# CALISTHENICS

*Becoming A Greek God – Shredded Through Calisthenics and Street Workout*

**Andrew Creager**

*Andrew Creager*

paraphrase any part or the content within this book without the consent of the author or copyright owner. Legal action will be pursued if this is breached.

# Table of Contents

# Introduction

When it comes to having a healthy lifestyle, some of us are a bit lazy. To be fair, we're probably all lacking in our physiques and our health. We all have work we can do to our bodies and its time for us to start making a difference. So let's get some things straight before we start. The first thing you want to know is why would you want to read this book and why is this book right for you?

The short answer is that I've done all of this myself. By changing my own life through working out, I can give you insight into the hardest part about overcoming what it is you're going to be facing on the road ahead. I'll give you all the proper advice and methods to change your body into something you can be proud of, whether you're overweight now or looking to actually put on the pounds. I'm going to give you everything you need to know for success.

I will give you key information to your success in exercising, as well as information that will help improve your health along the way. I will also give you information about how to accommodate your new workout regimen through diet, hydration, vitamins, minerals and spacing out your workout throughout a six-day regimen with a one-day break so that your muscles can regenerate.

Understanding how your body works in relation to the above mentioned items is crucial to your success as a whole, and your ability to carry through with your exercise plans on a long-term basis. You don't want to be one of those people who start an exercise program, begin making progress and then give up do you? No, you are in it for the long haul!

So let's not waste any more time and get started right away!

# Chapter 1
# Historical Calisthenics

Using bodyweight to increase physical strength is something that just comes naturally to both man and beast. Apes for example, develop physical strength constantly by swinging like Tarzan from one branch to another using one or both arms to propel their bodies. Some use both arms and legs to elevate their bodies off the ground when climbing up a tree. Some flap their wings to develop strength to fly in the air and stay there. The mere act of running and walking are already in and by themselves forms of bodyweight exercises – calisthenics.

The word is actually derived from – like many other modern English words – 2 Greek words. And those words are "kallos" – meaning beauty – and "sthenos" – meaning strength. Together, calisthenics means beautiful strength.

The word was believed to have been first utilized in Herodotus' chronicles on The Battle of Thermopylae around 480 BC. Based on this account, the "god-king" Xerxes' spies discovered that King Leonidas' army (remember the movie 300?) was practicing naked calisthenics.

Pausanias, a Greek geographer and traveller noticed that the original Olympic games athletes also trained in this beautiful art of strength. The historian Livy noted that the beautiful tradition of bodyweight calisthenics training continued even in the Romans' gladiator training camps. We may rationally conclude that every civilization and culture that ever existed in the world incorporated as part of its culture some form of bodyweight calisthenics training.

In India, physical fitness has long been an integral part of its culture and tradition – thousands of years to be more specific. The Indian culture has long been known for its various physical training instruments such as stone weights, maces, and heavy Indian clubs.

But bodyweight exercises – 2 in particular – were nonnegotiable in traditional training programs for Indian wrestlers: The dand or pushups and baithak or squats. When you look at their thousands of years old yoga postures – also called asanas – you'll find that many of the calisthenics practices that are being implemented today have a striking resemblance to them. It's even cooler when you realize that for the longest time in Indian culture, it was the warrior class who practiced these yoga asanas.

Steve Maxwell, America's first ever-certified Gracie Jiu-Jitsu trainer said in an interview that India practically started everything as we know it. He referred to the fact that Indian yogi rishis started the practice of meditation predated the Egyptian and Chinese cultures by 1,700 and 1,500 years, respectively. He also mentioned about how Gracie Jiu-Jitsu practitioners often talk about their martial art practically starting in India. And this particular form of martial arts is heavily reliant on bodyweight or calisthenics training.

It wasn't just Indians who were so into calisthenics ever since the world began. The Persians were also into it too. Their cultural tradition of Zurkaneh, which literally means

House of Strength, is known to have used systematic calisthenics or bodyweight exercises for thousands of years. And of course, who would miss out on the very famous Shaolin monks of China, eh? Since time immemorial, they've incorporated bodyweight calisthenics as an extensive means of developing their balance, agility and strength.

As civilization marched on towards more modern generations, bodyweight calisthenics continued to be very popular and well respected in terms of being a strength building method – even into the 19th and early 20th centuries. It was in the 19th century where strong men like Eugene Sandow – from whom the ultimate bodybuilding award, the Mr. Olympia, was named after – and Arthur Saxon have made physical strength the defining fitness characteristic. But around this time that the concept of weight-adjustable barbells and dumbbells was implemented, which announced the era of calisthenics' decline and seeming demise. And from the 20th century's 2nd half until today, calisthenics has been mostly dislodged and replaced by resistance training machines and contraptions like dumbbells, barbells and equipment like the Smith machine and lat pull-down, among others.

But despite their popularity, calisthenics continued to thrive, albeit in an underground fashion and away from the mainstream, particularly in prisons, martial arts houses, and military camps.

Thanks to the authors like Matt Furey, Brooks Kubik, Pavel Tsatsouline and Paul Wade and their books Combat Conditioning, Dinosaur Bodyweight Training, The Naked Warrior, and Convict Conditioning, respectively, bodyweight calisthenics is experiencing a rebirth – a mainstream one. In fact, that's one of the reasons you're holding this book now.

*Andrew Creager*

# Chapter 2

# Get a Physical

While this may seem trivial right now, it is important to get a complete physical before you begin an exercise program. This is because you want to ensure that your body is healthy enough for the workout regimen that you plan to partake in. The overall goal is to build a healthier, happier you and without ensuring that your body is healthy enough to withstand exercise, you cannot guarantee that this will be the outcome.

Let your doctor know at your physical that you plan to start an exercise program and what your goal is, whether it is to lose weight, gain muscle or just become healthier. Your doctor will perform a full physical examination and possibly run lab work to ensure that you do not have any underlying health condition that would prevent you from working out in a rigorous manner, or they may simply place limitations on your exercise routine due to weak ligaments or unstable joints. These limitations may change over time as you lose weight and strengthen your tendons and ligaments.

Once your doctor has the results of all of their tests, they can tell you what exercises are best for you. For example, if you have lived a sedentary lifestyle for a long period of time, your ligaments may be loose. Your doctor may recommend water aerobics to strengthen your ligaments without risking damage to them.

No matter what your doctor says, take their advice, they are trained professionals and have years of experience dealing with various clients who have been exactly where you are now.

Your doctor may recommend supplements to make up for vitamin or mineral deficiencies that you may have to help you along your way and will most likely review the basics of hydration with you to ensure that you are prepared to begin your exercise program. They may also be able to refer you to an excellent nutritionist that can help you get the most out of your exercise routine, especially if you are trying to lose weight, or bulk up.

## Do Not Begin an Exercise Program without Doctor Approval

It is important that you do not start any exercise program without the approval of your doctor. While exercise can increase your health it can also depreciate your health if you have a chronic, acute, or underlying condition that you are not aware of.

You should check in with your doctor regularly to ensure that you do not develop any vitamin deficiencies and that your health is improving instead of declining.

Very rarely an exercise program can cause a flare in an unknown medical condition that your doctor was unable to detect. Scheduling regular appointments with your doctor at the start of your exercise program will ensure that you do not fall victim to any secret your body may hold.Getting a physical done before joining an exercise program also helps people focus and individualize their fitness regime. A doctor helps a person decide on a more focused routine, suitable to that particular individual's health and fitness level.

Not only physically, a doctor can also help in preparing a person mentally for exercise and physical exertions.

Also one can determine whether their body is ready for fitness training or not. Getting physical exams and tests done can help with that. Having tests done before entering into a program and after it can help determine how much of an improvement in health has occurred. Both the pre and post program results can be compared with each other and checked for changes.

It is advised that before going for a physical, one should have a list of all the possible questions they might need to ask their doctor regarding the exercise program. And in case there is any problem, the doctor should be immediately alerted.

Here are a few problems that might be of concern:

-Discomfort, cramping or pain in the neck, chest or arms during any kind of physical activity.

-Blacking out or getting dizzy with physical stress

-Being short of breath when indulging in physical activity, or even before going to bed

-Ankle swelling

-A rapid heartbeat

-Any heart concerns that your doctor might have previously had

-Lower leg pain

Have a talk with your doctor about any of these problems or others as well. Potential risks, what to avoid, and what to do should be discussed in detail with the physician.

How can you decide if you should see your doctor?

One should go for a consultation if any of the following apply to them:

-Family history of cardiac diseases

-Diabetes or pre diabetes

-Have not exercised at all in the past three to four months.

-The person is above or between the ages of forty-five and

fifty-five.

-Currently smoking or has recently quit

-Overweight or obese

-Has high blood pressure or cholesterol above optimum levels

A consultation with the doctor can help avoid any negative impact of a physical activity on health. Athletes are also advised to go see physicians to avoid injuries and excel at sports and activities. Even if injury strikes, a physician is immediately summoned for assessment and can help with getting back into shape after the injury has been treated.

In today's digital age, the process has been further made easy. The Canadian Society for Exercise Physiology has developed a questionnaire for people deciding on seeing a doctor before embarking on an exercise regime. It is a very helpful tool called the Physical Activity Readiness Questionnaire (PAR-Q).

The kind of doctors that are recommended for consultations are:

-Physiatrists: These are doctors who specialize in training of bones, calf and neck muscles, as well as nerve movements. They are certified individuals who are eligible to treat back problems, strokes, Parkinson's disease, arthritis, and obesity. A physiatrist can work with restricted movements, pain, and even customize exercise routines to help a person get back in shape after an injury or medical problem. They can advise what kind of exercise to do and what to avoid depending on the condition of a person's health and fitness.

-Physical therapists: Help with bones and nerve relaxation. They can offer expertise in case of sprains, joint pains, and recovery from stroke or a heart attack. Their specialization can be in geriatrics or orthopedics.

-A to physical therapists: Help with the same kind of work, but only under the supervision of a physical therapist.

-Personal trainers: These are the fitness specialists who help train with the exercise regime. Their job is to oversee if a person is doing their routine properly and without any unnecessary exertions. Apart from that they also motivate, encourage, polish the skills of a person, tune up the person's form, and constantly push the person to do better. Trainers frequently change and shuffle routines to avoid monotony and boredom in exercise.

While licenses and certification is needed for therapists and doctors, fitness trainers require no particular formal accreditation. Just make sure that he or she is a recommended trainer and has done some courses or required training.

# Chapter 3
# How Muscles Work

There are two main types of muscles in your body that are developed through exercise and hard work. These muscles are the voluntary muscles and involuntary muscles.

Voluntary muscles are the ones that you can move freely wherever you want. When you are using your arms and legs, chewing food, or moving your head from side to side, you are using voluntary muscles. There is a darker side to muscles and that is that you do not have control over all of the muscles in your body.

Muscles like your heart and your lungs work through a system called the "autonomic nervous system." You have little to no control over these muscles. This makes living easier because you do not have to tell your heart to beat or your lungs to inhale; they do this on their own.

Whether muscles are voluntary or involuntary, you need to keep them strong. Just living everyday life is not enough to keep your involuntary muscles functioning at peak performance; you have to challenge them as well. That is why in this book, I recommend that as you are working on becoming ripped, you don't just focus on your voluntary muscles.

So how do you work on muscles that you have little to no control over? You put them in a situation where they are forced to work harder than ever before. Cardiovascular workouts cause your heart to pump faster and your lungs to inhale and exhale faster, in order to provide your body with enough blood and oxygen to sustain your muscles. While you are doing this, you are burning fat at astronomical speeds and you are increasing the visibility of the muscles that you are working so hard to build.

## Burning that Layer of Fat

Many people notice that as they workout and build muscle, a thin layer of fat stands between the muscles they have worked so hard to build, and the visibility of those muscles. This is especially true through the abdominal region.

Through cardiovascular workouts, you can burn this thin layer of fat, little by little.

## How Does Cardio Burn Fat?

The concept of a cardiovascular workout is to increase your core temperature in an effort to burn that hard to get to fat as well as increase the rate that your body is able to excrete fat deposits, rather than just rearranging them.

This fat is excreted through two main methods. The first method is through sweat, which is why your skin feels extremely oily after a heavy workout. The second method is your digestive system. As the fat breaks down, your blood stream carries it back to your intestines to be excreted through your digestive system.

*Andrew Creager*

# Chapter 4
# Factors to Monitor in Fat Burning

Apart from cardio and exercise routines, it is also very important to keep a check and balance on meals and maintain a healthy lifestyle. To burn fat it is also essential that special attention be given to nutrition and calorie intake. No amount of exercise will be able to help if you are indulging in heavy fatty foods and not monitoring diet properly.

You must drop your calorie intake by a significant amount to burn body fat. When a calorie shortfall occurs, the body makes use of the layer of fat that has been accumulated. That layer of fat is known as the adipose tissue. And when the body uses the fat to build up energy, the deposition of fat starts disappearing and it in turn makes the person grow leaner.

Calorie counting is not all to do with proteins and fibers. It has a lot do with mathematics and calculations as well. For example, if you are exercising regularly and are active, the calories you burn are approximately eighteen per pound of bodyweight or more.

On this basis, a two hundred pound person consumes about thirty six hundred calories daily. To start with reducing fat, one must focus on getting around a calorie intake of fourteen to sixteen per pound of bodyweight. That is about twenty-eight hundred to thirty-two hundred daily.

The easiest way of doing that is getting rid of all excess fat foods like butter, oil, and sugary products. Apart from that, keep a tab on little things like removing skin from chicken before eating it, and decrease red meat consumption. Substitute whole eggs with egg whites and avoid dairy products with whole milk.

Eat healthy by incorporating fish, fruits, fresh vegetables, and healthy fats such as nuts into your diet.

Hormonal control is also of utmost importance. Hormones also contribute to fat burning. Balancing the fat storing hormone can help melt body fat away. The ideal way to do this is to keep a tab on the carbohydrates that you are taking in.

Carbohydrates stimulate an insulin level that is a hormone that drives up the fat storing process. Eating fewer carbs help moderate insulin levels.

It is important to keep in mind that not all carbohydrates are equal. There are short fast digesting carbs that kick up insulin and long slow digesting carbs that have little effect on insulin levels. The short digesting carb foods are white bread, most cold cereals, any sweets, and white rice and potatoes.

Your diet should be maintained with slow digesting carbs that are found in whole-grain breads, oatmeal, sweet potatoes, and dry fruits. Try and consume meals with halved proportions of carbohydrates. If you are used to eating one piece of bread, try to eat only half. Similarly shorten meal portions.

Choose whole grained foods, non-white wheat with the exception of immediately after workout. Keep the carbs until up to or less than two grams per pound of bodyweight every day.

It's essential that one make a note of daily consumption of calories, fats, and proteins. Different types of calories have varied effects on the body. There are dietary fats that can be fattening since they are used in bodybuilding. It's actually more fattening than carbs and proteins.

Then there are carbs which are good for the body as well. They help fuel training and rigorous exercise. And as emphasized before, protein is the key. It builds muscle. Sometimes even fat can be utilized as it can help with hormones and vitamin absorption.

However if your aim is to look ripped, lean, and sport six pack abs, fats must be a bygone thing. Protein must be the focus. It builds muscle, boosts and increases metabolic function. According to the thermic effect of food, the body burns more calories in breaking down and processing protein than any other.

At least one gram of protein per pound of bodyweight is recommended every day. Proteins in diet are found in meats such as chicken, fish, egg whites and low-fat cottage cheese.

It is also recommended that you don't eat anything about

three hours before bed. This is advised because of the growth hormone (GH) that is released during the initial sleeps. This hormone is fat burning and sleeping on an empty stomach stimulates its function.

One very interesting supplement that monitors fat is Nitrous Oxide. It is known by many as the 'best fat burning supplement' on the market. When taken before training, it increases blood flow, pumps muscles, and helps generate tissues and fast metabolism.

An arginine based and a five to ten gram dosage before going to bed can help surge GH levels and burn fat faster.

When maintaining a fitness routine, to properly get rid of excess fats, it is advised that you eat small meals every day up to six to eight times.

Eat more but eat healthy. It is said that eating frequently leads more muscle tissue being generated instead of the energy being converted to fat. Eat six to eight times a day spaced between two to three hours. Don't extend the break of more than three hours because than the body will experience a starvation mode and overeating is bound to occur.

It's very important that while keeping a check on your eating habits, you don't eat too little. After exercising, the body burns fat and the process is hindered if the body has no energy and is bordering on starvation.

Consume adequate proteins, sometimes even available in powder shape, fast digesting carbs, and sports drinks such as Gatorade.

Finally, when monitoring all of this, take special care that when you are training, you only go until a point when you are beat up. Getting exhausted and going overboard in the gym or during exercise is not advised. Serious fat loss requires muscle mass and if you burn yourself out too fast, it impedes the process.

Train intensely and as much as you like, just don't go on for excessive periods and longer than say an hour and a half in one session.

# Chapter 5
# Points of Interest

Before we actually start talking about the exercises that you should be dedicating your time to, I'm going to give you a few insights into what you should be paying attention to in order to obtain the best possible results and experience when it comes to working out.

## Physical and Mental Benefits

The physical and mental benefits that you experience from exercise completely outweigh the benefits of any medication or supplement that you can take to lose weight. It has also proven its worth in treating anxiety, depression and a wide array of other mental illnesses that are commonly treated with toxic medications.

An exercise program is recommended by many therapists,

psychiatrists, and group therapists in order to treat various disorders. Some medical professionals recommend a combination of medication therapy and an exercise program. Over time, many patients have shown a decrease in symptoms requiring a lower dose of medication than they originally started on.

## Go to a Gym

The first point that I want to make with you is that the gym can be your best friend when you are trying to get into shape, lose weight and develop a healthier lifestyle. Gyms are more affordable than ever and you shouldn't be afraid of spending ten to thirty dollars a month for your health and well being. While you may think this is expensive, the investment will be worth it because it provides all the resources that you will need to accomplish your exercises and meet your goals. Plus, gyms are going to give you plenty of free information and motivation. You have a chance to watch those you seek to emulate and how they utilize their bodies and their form. Plus, it gives you an environment and an atmosphere that is truly motivating. When you are exercising using the weight of your body, having people around you that are accustomed to performing the exercises can really help you although this isn't obligatory.

When you work out at home, you have the ability to be lazy, lie to yourself, and overestimate what you have done. You also have the ability to slack off and not work your body as hard as you can. With people watching, there is more of a chance that you will push your body harder than you would in private. In a gym, your brain tells you to push your body harder to keep up with the people that you want to emulate.

## A Gym is Not Mandatory

While a gym can help you to develop healthy habits, it is not mandatory. You can easily workout at home if you are self-conscious. It is important that you do not sacrifice your form just because you are at home. Utilize workout videos that show the proper form for each exercise and always choose videos that allow you to work at your own pace.

Never jump into a "hardcore" program like P90x when you first start out. Choose programs that are at the beginner's level and work your way up from there. After you have mastered the beginner's program, you can move to the intermediate program and work your way up to an advanced program.

Even if you are working on a video that is a specific level, you can always slow your program down by going at your own pace to prevent injury or complete exhaustion. If you notice that you are extremely weak or sore after a workout, do not push yourself as hard the next time you exercise.

## Form

It is more important to have form than lift massive amounts of weight. If you use your body properly for the moves that you make, you will keep everything intact and everything healthy. Making one wrong move can put you out of commission for weeks, if not months. Keeping your body in form is important. Thus, respect the way that exercises are performed and do not be tempted to push yourself beyond your own personal limits. It's also a good idea to check with your doctor to be sure that it's okay to be doing these exercises given your current state of health.

If you do have health problems, your doctor may

recommend alternative exercises to help you lose weight and gain the physical form that you are looking for. Over time, as your health improves, your doctor may allow you to do more and more exercises.

## Weights

For many people who are new to working out, weights are unnecessary. It is because your body weight can provide enough resistance to burn calories and build muscle. Weights are for people who have been working out for quite a while and have developed enough strength that their body weight no longer provides an adequate workout. The added weight that you use will help you to increase your muscle mass as well as decreasing the amount of body fat that you carry around on a regular basis. We will cover more on weight lifting later.

## Supplements

The only supplements that I'm going to endorse for you here is Creatine and a multi-vitamin. The reason I'm going to limit my recommendations to a multi-vitamin and Creatine will become pretty obvious over time. Everyone should take a multi-vitamin daily to help enhance his or her dietary intake. Our diets are lacking in basic essentials and we just can't fit everything that we need to into our meals.

Creatine on the other hand has been under the scrutiny of scientists and officials for generations. It has come out on top and the results that it provides are without a doubt miraculous. You can do a lot of great work with the help of Creatine and it's the number one supplement that you'll want to put in your body. We will cover the benefits of this wonderful supplement later in this book.

## Nutrition

This is the final point I want to emphasize to you in this chapter. Nutrition is the law of the land when it comes to changing your body shape. Working out is essentially tearing down your muscle and rebuilding it stronger and with better materials. Nutrition comes down to simply replacing what you eat now with better foods. A cross section of foods that gives you the balance of goodness that you need is important. Make it a slow and steady transition so that it's not too much of a system shock to you. Take it slow; make pragmatic changes to your life so that you can start living a better life.

So what do you do about the snacks you crave throughout the day? You know, the ones you aren't supposed to have but your belly is giving you a heads up that it needs something to entertain itself. I will teach you about negative calorie foods so that even though you are dieting, you don't feel like you are starving yourself at any point in time.

## Hydration

Hydration is one of the most important aspects of working out. If you do not stay hydrated you can develop serious health complications, including cramps and long-term organ damage from chronic dehydration. I will talk about various measures you can take in order to prevent dehydration as well as the accommodations that must be made to the standard hydration rules in order to accommodate an exercise regimen.

With those points out of the way, let's get started on the real stuff and break down the ins and outs of the topics I have touched on in this chapter and the previous chapters.

*Andrew Creager*

# Chapter 6
# Preparing for a Workout

## Pre-workout Meals

Research shows that a pre-workout meal can help increase your energy level during a workout. This meal should be high in healthy carbohydrates and should be consumed at least three hours before your workout. After this meal, the only thing you should ingest is water or a sports drink.

As with any physical activity, eating too close to your workout can cause cramps, nausea, light-headedness, fatigue, and vomiting. This is because as you work out, your muscles contract rapidly, heating up your core temperature to a point that your body is not used to, especially with food sitting in your stomach.

It is okay to eat a meal an hour after working out, but you

should never eat a meal or consume dairy products within three hours of starting your workout.

In order to ensure that you do not injure yourself during exercise, regardless of what exercise you plan to perform, you should ensure that you properly stretch. Failing to stretch causes you to begin exercising using rigid muscles. If your muscles are rigid, as in, not in a position where they can be considered flexible, you can cause yourself serious injury.

Stretching prepares muscles for exercise in many different ways. First, it helps to bring extra oxygen to your muscles, which prepares them for movement. It also helps release lactic acid that has built up from living a sedentary lifestyle.

Stretching also helps improve the flexibility of the muscles you are using and loosens up the ligaments and tendons in preparation for the difficulty they will be soon be facing. When working out, you want your muscles to be loose and you want to ensure that they have free range of motion, which dramatically reduces the risk of injury.

Your body goes through a lot while you are exercising so preparing properly is important. While stretching is important, warming up is just as important. We will cover warming up later in this chapter.

## Risks of Failing to Stretch

Failing to stretch puts you at risk for multiple injuries. You could pull a muscle, tear a tendon,  or even a ligament. Many people have experienced an injury that has plagued them on a long-term basis due to failing to stretch. Most people end up needing expensive physical therapy, just to live a normal life that is free from pain and pain pills.

More extensive injuries could result in necessary surgery to repair the injury site. This surgery is expensive and very painful. Many patients report that even after surgery, they do not regain full function of the injury site.

The majority of people who have participated in clinical research studies after an exercise injury find that any form of exercise aggravates their pre-existing condition. This means, that if you do not take care of your body before, during, and after workouts, you may injure yourself to the point where you will no longer be able to exercise. By failing to follow this advice, you may have to give up that ripped, perfect physique that you have been dreaming of your entire life.

If this does not scare you into stretching properly, nothing will. You only get one body, so why not make the most of it and develop the body of your dreams safely and effectively.

## Warming Up

After stretching, you should always warm up your muscles. This is the second part in preparing them for the trials of your workout. Failing to warm up poses the same risks as not stretching, but also increases the risk that you will develop severe cramps during the workout.

Warming up can involve anything that gets your muscles moving and your heart rate up. Many people choose to stretch, jog for 10 minutes, and then stretch again before a workout. This helps properly prime your muscles for the punishment that they are going to receive from your exercise program.

## Cooling Down

Most people experience pain and soreness after exercising,

especially if they are doing it right. In order to reduce the amount of soreness that you experience, you should properly cool down by jogging and then complete your workout with a full set of stretches.

The purpose of cooling down and stretching after a workout is actually pretty simple. Just like any other item that breaks down, muscles release a chemical as they are worked. This chemical is called lactic acid. After you finish working out and your muscles begin to cool down on their own, this lactic acid begins to build up in your system. If it is allowed to stay in your body and is not directed to an exit point through your blood stream, it can result in excessive soreness and long-term tenderness in your joints.

Cooling down properly and stretching after exercise helps to release the lactic acid from your muscles and joints into your blood stream. It is then carried to your digestive system for normal excretion.

So if you want to ensure that you do not develop excessive soreness, tenderness and pain, you should follow the following system:

1.    Warm Up – It starts warming up your muscles in

preparation for your workout. Warm-up by getting your blood pumping and increasing your heart rate to at least 160 beats per minute. This will ensure that your cardiovascular system and lungs are ready for the workout they are going to endure. This can also reduce the risk of your lungs feeling as though they are on fire from increasing your respiratory rate too rapidly.

2.    Exercise – Complete your workout to the best of your ability, pushing your body only to a point that is comfortable. Keep in mind that exercise is painful, but I cover the signs of overdoing your exercise routine.

3.    Cool Down – Cooling your body down slowly is extremely important. You will want to ensure that you cool down for at least 10 minutes before you begin your stretching.

4.    Stretch Again – Stretching after exercise releases the lactic acid that has built up in the muscles that you have worked out. This will reduce the amount of soreness that you experience in your muscles and joints.

Following these directions will keep your body in top shape throughout your workout and after.

## Protein Follow-up

After working out, your muscles need protein in order to rebuild themselves. It is important that you eat a meal that is rich in protein, or drink a protein shake.

You may want to allow your core temperature to cool down before drinking a protein shake, as many of them have a milk base and a high core temperature can cause you to feel sick to your stomach.

*Andrew Creager*

# Chapter 7

# Separating Your Workout

While it may seem tempting to take care of your workout all at once, this can leave you extremely fatigued and leave your body in a malnourished state. Focusing on one aspect of your body at a time is ideal if you want to build the perfect physique. Because of this, your workout should be spread out through multiple days and should be developed to suit your needs.

## Hiring a Personal Trainer

While it may seem impractical at first, hiring a personal trainer to begin your exercise program is one of the best ways to ensure that you do not cause yourself any injury. Exercising is a dangerous sport, but it is necessary for your health and well being. Failing to have the proper form can cause serious injury. A personal trainer can assist you in learning the proper form and in developing an exercise routine that will prevent injury, provide maximum results, and show you the proper form for every exercise that you plan to do.

## Personal Trainers Are Not Expensive

In comparison to developing a long-term injury and paying the associated medical bills, a personal trainer is extremely inexpensive. You may not think so at first, but if you have ever pulled a muscle, torn a ligament, or over-extended an extremity, you know how painful it can be. A personal trainer's job is to prevent you from harming yourself, or the people around you as you exercise. Think of it as a safety lesson before you decide to jump straight into a hardcore workout.

## Separating Your Workout by Day

It may seem strange to refer to your workout as leg day, core day, and arm day and so on, but this is an important aspect in developing a healthy body. When you work out, you put a lot of strain on your body. It takes a great deal of time for the muscles that you have broken down to regenerate and become stronger. This is why working your entire body out daily is an extremely bad idea.

Because you want to increase your health, you should focus on one aspect of your body per day, giving the strained and broken down muscles time to heal before you tear them down again.

In this book, I recommend working out for six days and taking the seventh day to rest all of your muscles.

## Why Take a Day to Rest

Many people jump into a workout regimen and feel that they have to exercise seven days a week in order to see results. Typically, these people are the ones who develop short term and long-term injuries.

When you are working out, you are breaking down the muscle that already exists. Essentially, you are turning it into mush, which is why it typically hurts the next day. Failing to give your muscles time to heal after they have been broken down can result in permanent damage to the affected muscle.

When you perform an exercise, you are not using a single

muscle group; you are using multiple muscle groups. There is no way to isolate a single muscle group, therefore you must give your body a break at some point to avoid inadvertently damaging a muscle that you don't even known you are working. The only way to ensure that you give your body the proper amount of time to heal is to take a full 24 hours to rest all of your muscles.

If you are working out on a regular basis, and you are short on time, you may need to take two days off in order to allow your body time to regenerate. This is a judgment call for each individual person and you may need to adjust this according to your body, your medical conditions, and your personal stamina level.

## Determining If Your Workout Is Too Strenuous

Feeling sore the day after a workout is normal. You basically just tore apart a muscle in order to make it stronger. However, there is a point where your body warns you that you are on the verge of overdoing it, or that you have already overdone it.

The day after a workout your body should feel sore, but the

pain should be bearable. It feels more like the muscles are extremely warm and they may feel a little tight the next day from any excess lactic acid that was not released after your workout. There are some things you should not feel after a workout including:

- Sharp pains

- Unbearable aching

- Debilitating pain

- Inability to lift items (for example, if you cannot lift a full coffee cup)

- Extreme tenderness around your joints

- Limits in your range of motion

- Inability to move a joint

- Swelling

- Redness

- Nausea

- Feeling as though you have the flu

If you feel any of these symptoms, you should go to your doctor or urgent care right away.

If at any point you have over exerted your muscles, you should take a few days off of your exercise plan to allow it to heal, unless your doctor recommends that you avoid exercising for a longer period of time.

If the problem persists, you may require x-rays or immobilization of the area that is affected. During the time that you are unable to exercise, you should review what went wrong. Did you ignore your form? Did you overexert your muscles? Did you try to do too many repetitions? Maybe you tried to lift too much weight?

Once you have determined what went wrong with your exercise on the day of your injury, you can properly adjust your workout to prevent the injury from reoccurring or getting worse.

# Chapter 8
# Street Workout

Let's begin this by defining what a street workout is. You might have heard the term a lot in recent times. It is a fad gaining rapid popularity.

It is a physical activity that is mostly done outdoors. Like in parks, open grounds, and vast areas. It is a combination of calisthenics and athletics. Calisthenics are exercises that usually combine movement skills with sport activities. And athletics are sports.

A typical routine of a street workout consists of push-ups, pull-ups, squats and dips. One of the main attractive features of a street workout is the fact that it is free and promotes a healthy lifestyle in an easy way.

For beginners, it is easy to get going with it. It involves a basic warm up and stretch to flex the body a little.

These workout routines involve working with the abdominal muscles, legs, and chest as well.

Some of the basic exercises include:

- Lunges

- L-Sit Hangs

- Push Ups

- Chin Ups

- Dips

- Sit Ups

- Normal Grip Pull Ups

- Squats

The thing to remember is that you need to only push yourself according to the capability of the body. Take a rest of thirty to forty seconds between each exercise and maybe up to a minute if you are a total beginner.

A few more of the focus exercises are abs, legs, biceps, and chest.

## Abdominal Muscles

1.      Start with thirty Seconds of Mountain Climbers and Leg Raises. Then repeat.

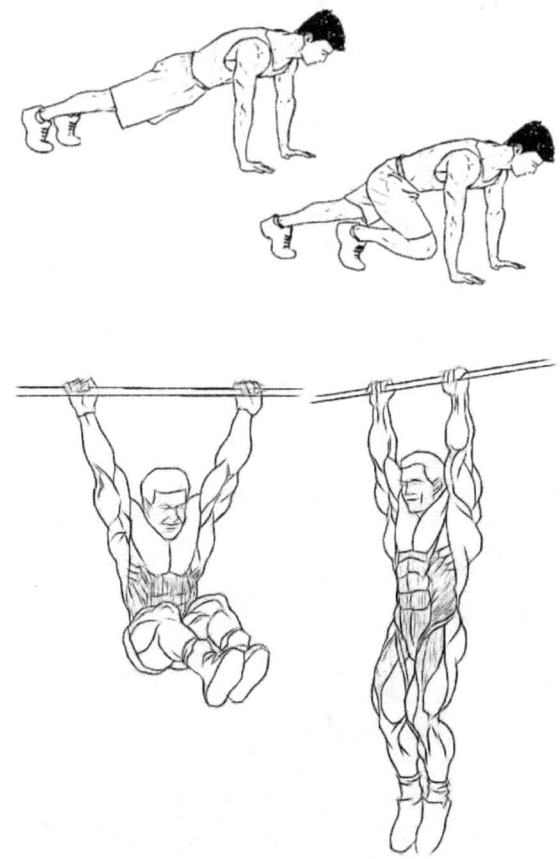

2. Do ten to fifteen seconds of Leg Raises.

3. Then go back to Mountain Climbers for about thirty to forty seconds.

Follow that with another 15 seconds of Leg Raises.

4. Revert back to thirty seconds of Mountain Climbers.

5. Go for a hundred Flutter Kicks.

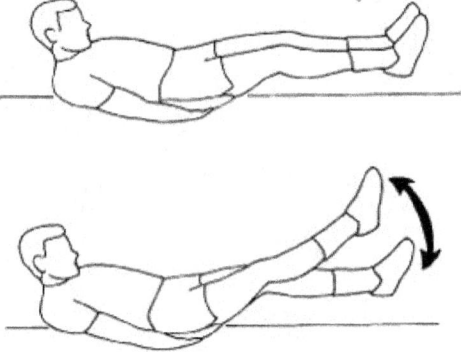

6. Finish off with Mountain Climbers and Crunch holds.

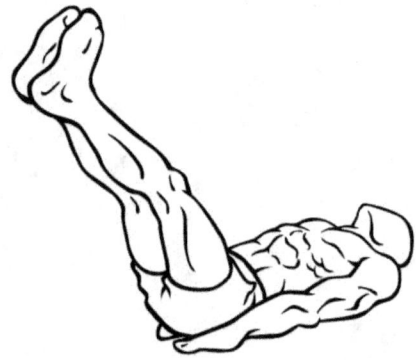

It is recommended that you do three rounds with rest in between rounds depending on your level.

Yes, it does indeed look like a hard workout routine but do try doing it and if it really is too hard then you should lower the repetitions and increase breaks of seconds for every exercise and work your way up until you can finish this abs workout routine.

It does give sure shot results and soon you will be sporting abs that will be the envy of many.

This one is a more advanced workout routine for people who have accustomed their bodies to working out.

This is a full body workout combining leg muscles, arms and back.

**Workout:**

Start with Burpees doing a half maximum number of repetitions of this exercise.

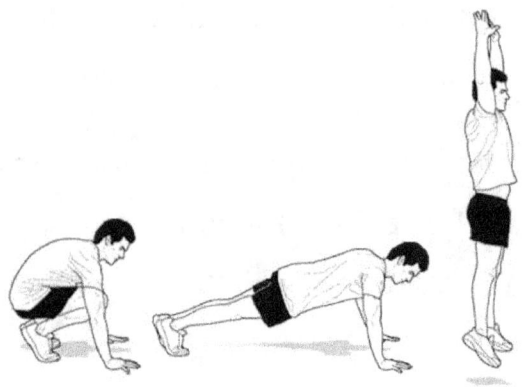

Then go on to Pull Ups and continue with twenty of them. Mix it up with three ab hits on each repetition; it is advised that this is done with a partner.

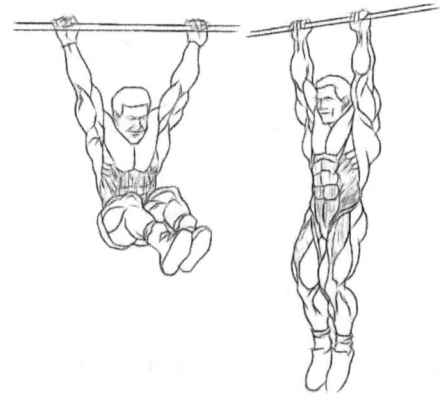

Go on to Push Ups. If you think that this is easy, think again. These thirty Push Ups need to be done with someone on your back! This set also requires a partner.

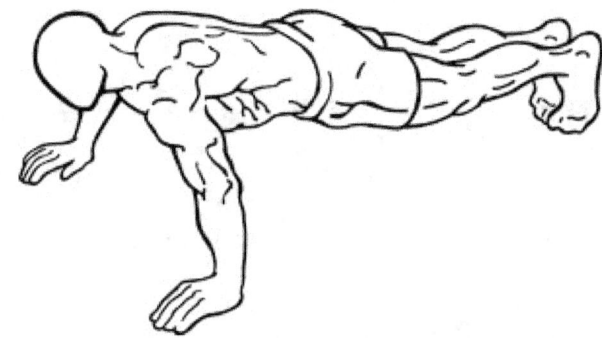

Then there comes the Squat Frog Jumps. Each repetition will consist of doing a high jump squat and then when you get in the low squat position again, attempt a frog jump. Repeat.

Follow that up with some leg raises, usually beginners will do about 3 – 5, while the more trained and advanced will go between 10 – 20.

Finish off with maximum Burpees.

It does seem like a hard one to get through. But try to maintain focus and break less. Finish the repetitions in one go before going on to break. This will help with time management and make it easy to get the routine done.

**Leg Routine**

Squats

Start with basic squats which when done correctly are a good way to start. Keep in mind that before starting with the routine you are properly warmed up.

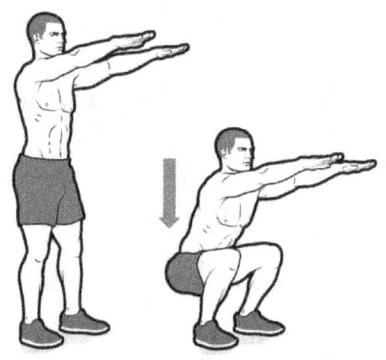

Calf Raises

Do these in variations. Don't just go on doing a single type of calf raises. This will increase focus on other muscles as well.

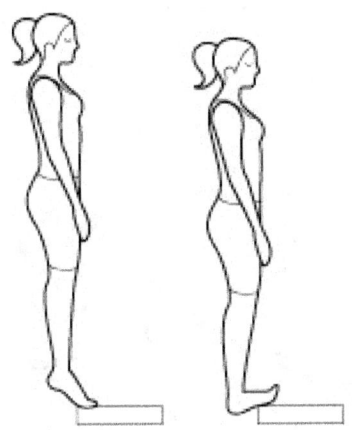

Pistol Squats

Not everyone can do it. So this is just optional. These are the same exercise as normal squats, but with one leg. Hold onto a wall with one hand if you need to maintain your balance.

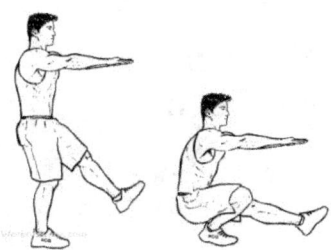

Low Squat Holds

This will be the single steady part of the workout routine that will keep the tension in the muscles and make you experience a burning sensation after you do all the other exercises.

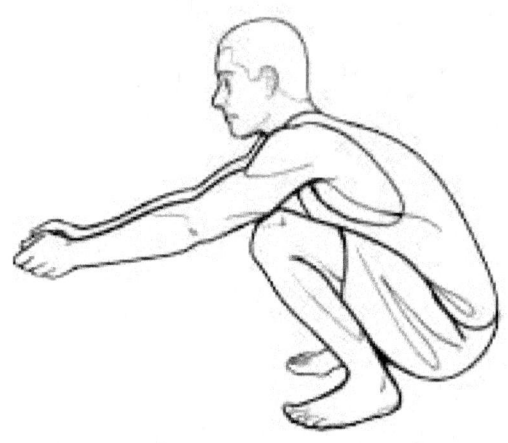

Legs Bodyweight HIIT Routine:

This routine has six exercises that you will need to fit in one cycle. After each exercise you should take a break of maximum fifteen seconds and go to the next exercise until you finish the entire cycle. If you are more advanced and want to take this as a challenge; take no or very little rest between exercises.

But if you what you are looking for is a quick workout then take up to one minute of rest between exercises or cycles.

1. Start by attempting twenty Lunges (Do not miss out on

the warm up)

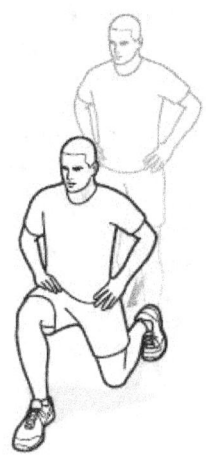

2. Then proceed to twenty seconds of sprinting

3. Follow that up by seven to ten Burpees. In the middle try and fit in a minute of Rope Skipping to cool down a bit.

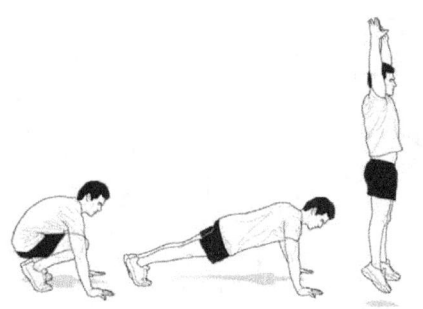 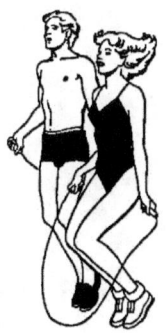

Then do twenty to thirty proper form Squats.

And finish by again repeating the second step. Sprint.

The numbers given in the exercise routine can be changed to adapt to one's current fitness level and body capacity. However it should be noted that this is a HIIT (High Intensity Interval Training). You should feel your body getting beat and the burn in your muscles that comes from doing certain exercises.

Pull Up bar Routine:

Get on a bar and try to do as many Wide Pull Ups as you can.

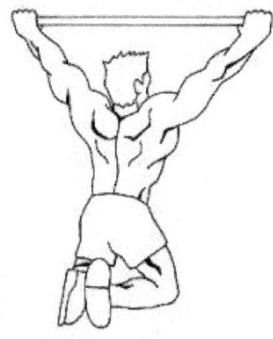

Then without dropping yourself from the bar, try and get into a narrow pull up position and pull up. Now attempt to hold that static position for as long as you can.

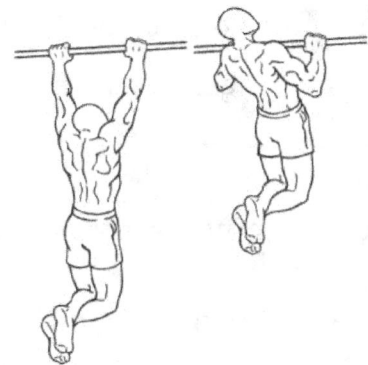

This is a strictly if you can thing. While on the bar, try to do at least twenty leg raises. That can do wonders with your abs and your forearms.

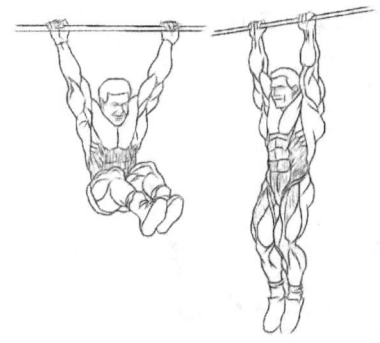

And now, when you are done with all these bar exercises, get down and do the maximum amount of push-ups.

This workout routine is to focus on your endurance levels. Because of that you should make sure that a proper warm up has been done before the actual workout set. It makes a marked difference. After you are done with one set of the above workout go for a longer pause than usual so that your muscles can recover.

Give yourself five to ten minutes after each set.

These are some of the street workouts that are known to produce maximum results. They have all been devised by workout pros and can be attempted by both beginners and people who are more advanced in their workout regimes.

Now let's go on to another topic. This is actually a question raised by people, who argue why a street workout might be better than a gym workout.

Look at it as a debate.

If one is to list the pros of street workouts, they would be freedom, no rules, can be done anywhere and everywhere, needs no money and no equipment. A person has creative freedom to do the exercise in whatever way he or she may like.

Looking at gyms, one can say that there is motivation that comes from paying for it and from trainers. Programs can be constructed to suit one's form and fitness. It works for all seasons and weather and helps one stay active.

Each of them has their own advantages and one can never say which one is better. It is simply left to one's own personal choice.

Street workouts are gaining more and more followers worldwide as more and more people lose weight and have their lives turned around.

*Andrew Creager*

# Chapter 9
# Calisthenics

As said before, Calisthenics are exercises that have much to do with the motor skills of a person. It is in essence, body weight training. These exercises aim to increase body resistance, flexibility, and strength through movements.

Common exercises are pushing, pulling, bending, jumping, or swimming. All of these have to make use of the body's weight for resistance. They are usually done with a follow up of stretches, both pre and post workout.

When performed with consistency and vigor, these can do wonders for the body.

Increased agility, prominence in shape, muscle buildup, and better co-ordination are just some of the various benefits of the exercise. It is often known to be done in groups and synchronized movements to increase focus and discipline.

Calisthenics has programs in schools across the globe. It is also known to be endorsed by the U.S army as a basic physical evaluation test.

The word Calisthenics is derived from the two ancient Greek words, 'Kalos' meaning beauty and 'Sthenos' which means strength. It gained prominence since the early nineteenth century and today has been incorporated in the rapidly growing Street Workout regime.

As a sport it can be conducted within that range, where athletes compete against one another by comparing body weight and body strength. There is a World Street Workout & Calisthenics Federation (WSWCF), which is based in Latvia.

It organizes the annual National Championships in up to fifty different countries (as of 2015) and hosts the World Championships.

Common exercises include Lunges, Planks, Jumping Jacks, Crunches, Push-ups, Pull-ups, Dips, Hyperextensions, and

Leg Raises.

Calisthenics can be done in areas outdoors and in parks. A fun way of doing some of these exercises is to be at a Jungle Gym.

Now let's move on to some of the effective Calisthenics exercises that are going to help keep that weight off.

Starting with the basics and how to do them:

**Various pull-ups**

An overhead bar (also called a chin-up bar) is grasped using a shoulder-width grip. Lift the body up, chin level with the bar, and keep the back straight throughout. The bar remains in front of the person at all times. Slowly return to starting position in a steady controlled manner.

This is good for the lats or upper back muscles, as well as the forearms. An underhand grip variation or chin-up helps both the back and biceps.

**Pushups**

These are exercises that focus on the core area of the body. Explained further downwards, they are performed facing down towards the floor, palms flat against it with the toes standing up against it as well. The arms are used to lift the body. Chest, shoulders, and triceps are built with this exercise.

## Squats

As explained later in detail, squats are basically movements of legs and thighs that help strengthen hamstrings and calves.

## Various dips

This is done to focus on your whole upper-body. Feet are crossed with either foot in front and the body is lowered. Line the elbows with the shoulders. Then push up until the arms are fully extended, but without locking the elbows. These are done with bars.

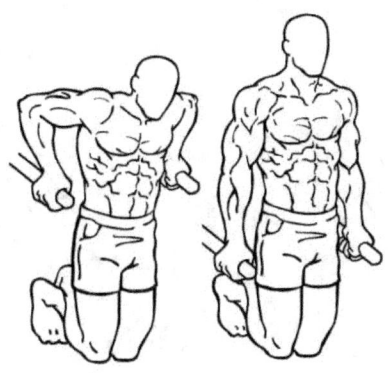

## Ab exercises

There are several exercises to maintain body weight in the abdomen. Having a strong core is essential in calisthenics.

## Hyperextensions

Performed in a prone (chest down, back up) position on the ground, the person is required to raise the legs, arms, and upper body off the ground.

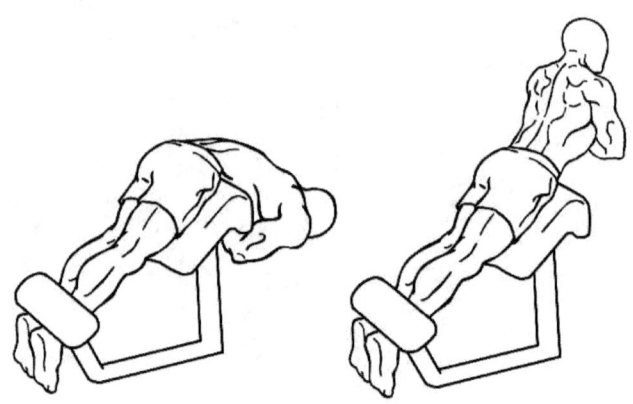

For beginners, it can only be said that they need to do the exercises correctly. It is critical that you keep a check on your motions when doing the routine. Many people give up after a month or so as they complain of not getting results. That's because they are not really moving the right way.

Getting results takes hard work and patience. Just don't give up. Increase the sets and timings as you progress further. If you feel your body adapting to the exercise, toughen the regime. Vice versa, if there is a part that needs working on, double the effort.

Keep yourself motivated. Look at people who are fit, watch videos, and be aware of your own self. Get a good look at yourself and know which areas to work on.

If you are overweight, start a diet and do some cardio training to drop the weight along the way. Stretching is also crucial to the workout. Do it after and before performing calisthenics exercises.

For total beginners, it is suggested that they attempt beginner exercises before.

These include Chin-ups with the assistance of a resistance band, including negative pull ups, dips with the band, dips behind back, and knee push-ups. Do this routine three to four times a week until you get stronger and familiar with these workouts. Go on for about a month or two and then change to the basic exercises mentioned above.

For more advanced people, the basic exercises include:

Chest

**Push ups**

This is to build your upper bod. It works your pectorals, triceps, and anterior deltoid. For this exercise work up to high rep range and then add weight.

If someone can only do ten to twelve body weight push-ups,

then they shouldn't add weight and work on getting their ranges up. Then start to add weight gradually. Enlist the help of a partner and get them to stand next to you pushing down on your back (lightly or hard depending on strength).

## Chest Dip

You can easily set up two couches or two chairs together. Be creative with whatever you have, and make sure you are safe doing it. A bad setup can lead to instant injury, so be careful with how you set this up.

## Incline Push ups

Perform a regular push up and then elevate your feet with a bench, bed, chair, etc. This will target more of the upper pectorals and help develop those.

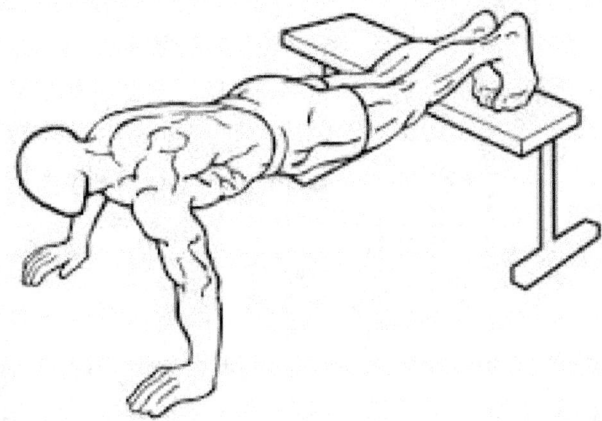

Back

## Chin-ups

This is one of the best builders for the back. It develops the lats, more than most exercises, and can result in a nice strong back. Look for a place where you can do these safely. It should be sturdy. If you can attempt these for a high amount of ranges then get someone to push down on your shoulders while you are doing it for added benefit.

## Underhand Chin-ups

This is almost the same exercise just with a different grip. Most feel quite comfortable doing the underhand grip. You will be able to lift more when you do these, so use resistance if required.

## Hyperextensions

This exercise is good for strengthening the lower back. Another way to perform this exercise is on the edge of a bed or chair with someone holding your feet so your place is solid and will not result in a fall. Make sure you do this exercise safely; injuries can occur in case of any mishap.

Thighs

## Squats

For this exercise you don't need weight. Go all the way down and back up. When you need resistance, get a partner to hold your shoulders and apply pressure downward. This is great for developing the quadriceps.

## Lunges

Just focus on getting low on this exercise and high repetition sets. It is hard to add weight. It is great for building chest muscles.

-Split Single Leg Squats

This exercise is better without weight and a prominent developer of the quadriceps. You can put your leg up on a chair, on a step, and anything you can find that is steady, solid, and safe.

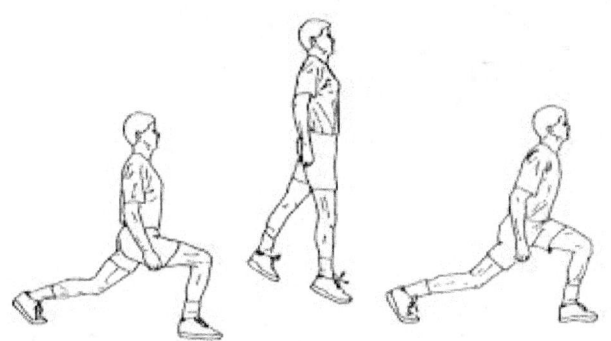

## Glute Ham Raise

This exercise is really good for the hamstrings. You will need a strong partner to support you on this exercise that is basically like a hyperextension, with the difference being that you have to curl your leg when you go up.

Abdominal:

## Crunches

Just basic crunches are all you need to work your abdominal area.

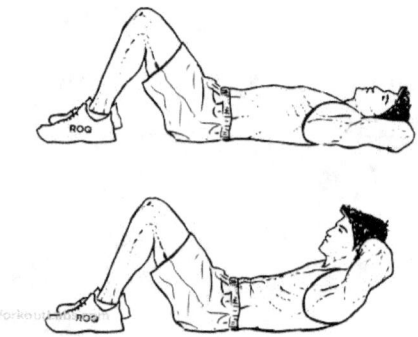

Calves:

## Calf Raises

Do calf raises on a step or any block that is solid and steady.

Calisthenics are amazing for weight free, hassle free, and muscle building exercises. They are a combination of all such healthy exercises that promote flexibility, discipline, help get rid of excessive weight and increase endurance levels.

And they are not even boring. Mix in a couple of exercise routines, adjust timings and repetitions, and you will be enjoying yourself in a few days' time.

# Chapter 10
# Weights are Unnecessary

For many people, especially those who are just starting out, weights are an unnecessary accessory. This is because their body weight provides enough resistance in a standard exercise setting. If you have not worked out for several years, you may need to adjust simple exercises to reduce the amount of body weight you are supporting. For example, if you are not able to do 10 pushups, you may want to do pushups on your knees.

If you do choose to use weights, especially free-weights, choose lightweights to start out with and work your way up slowly as your body becomes accustomed to the strain.

Progressing through your workout too fast can dramatically increase your chances of developing an injury. Listen to your body and allow it to pave the way to becoming a healthier, happier, ripped version of your old self.

Many people who develop injuries early on in their exercise career do so because they overestimate the amount of weight they can safely lift repetitively. Lifting too much weight at a time, especially when you are not accustomed to lifting weights can cause serious, long-term injury.

I recommend holding off on using weights until you become more familiar with your body's capabilities and the movements necessary to complete each exercise. You should also ensure that you have developed a fair amount of flexibility and an adequate range of motion to accommodate the exercise while supporting the extra weight that is involved.

When you are ready for weights, start out with two to three pound weights and work your way up as you develop comfort and control over the weights over an extended period of time.

After you have become accustomed to the weights, you can modify the exercise in various ways. You can do this by increasing elevation, decreasing elevation, adding a yoga ball to your weight lifting routine and even increasing the amount of weight you lift.

## Yoga Balls

While yoga balls technically do not fall under the category of weights, they can still be dangerous for those who are new to exercising. It is not advisable to perform any exercise that relies on you being in a position that causes strain while using a yoga ball as the main support. It is definitely not advisable for someone who is new to working out to lift weights while using a yoga ball.

A yoga ball does have a purpose for those who are new to exercising. This benefit is the ability to build posture and core strength. In order to do this, you do not need any special equipment or any special exercise maneuvers. Simply sitting on an exercise ball at work or while you are watching television can help to strengthen your core muscles and improve posture. It also helps to strengthen your back and reduce the risk of injury when you are exercising.

After you have been lifting weights for a long time, you may want to use a yoga ball to help work your core while you are lifting weights. You may also want to use it to prop your feet up while doing pushups in order to increase the amount of weight that you use as resistance in a simple exercise.

# Chapter 11

# If You're an Absolute Beginner

If you're just new to calisthenics or exercising in general, it would be wise for you to hold your horses and begin with basic street workout routines first. Why? Going all gung-ho and full-speed ahead with harder and more advanced routines significantly increases your risks for both burning out (dropping the endeavor altogether) and injuring yourself. Remember, you want to make fitness and health a lifetime thing, not a flash-in-the-pan state.

## Patience

Rome wasn't built in a day and it will be the same for that dream body of yours. Be patient. The fittest men you've seen who've done and continue to do calisthenics street workouts have been at it for quite some time now and as such, you'll also have to pay your dues to get to their level of fitness.

Many beginners start with guns a-blazin' and with all the spunk of the Energizer bunny who just downed a large can of Monster energy drink hoping to get fit and ripped in a month's time. Unfortunately, their over-zealousness often leads to burn out or worse, injuries. It's because impatience is the precursor to improper form and working out too hard.

## Proper Form

Speaking of, one of the worst mistakes most beginners make, which I'm sure you'll want to avoid, is performing the exercises with improper form. Many people drop out of their calisthenics street workout routines after a few short months due to lack of results, primarily from doing the exercises wrong. By sticking to the basics first, you'll be able to concentrate on getting it right the first time, which will maximize your desired results from your workouts. And if you see more results then you'll be encouraged to continue and experience more results. This will become a powerful upward spiral into even better fitness. So if you're torn between being able to complete the number of reps in the workout routines in this book and being able to exercise proper form, go for the latter. It's always better to do less of the right thing than more of the wrong one. Believe me, going to great lengths just to master proper form can save you more time, effort, and potential injuries.

## Intensity

Another child of impatience is doing exercises at a very high intensity that can be too much for one's current level of fitness. Getting ripped is a combination of passionate commitment to doing the exercises as well as wisdom. A brainless passionate commitment just won't cut it, or worse, can even do you more harm than good.

For the most part, especially in the beginning, you'll need to exercise at a moderate intensity. Low intensity workouts are too easy and they won't lead to better strength and fitness. High intensity – if done so often – increases your risk of burning out or getting injured and as such, high intensity street workouts are best incorporated into your routine on an interval basis and not as the norm if you'd like to last long. Moderate intensity gives you just enough physical stress that will allow you to enjoy continuously healthy improvements in physical strength and fitness.

So how do you know if you're trying too hard? One way is the talk test. If you can barely talk while exercising, that's too hard. If you can talk normally, then it's low intensity. If you can still talk but with some difficulty, that's moderate. Go for moderate.

Physically, you'll know if you're exercising too hard or soft by how your body feels afterwards, particularly the next day. If you always experience regular body aches, then it's a sign that you may be overdoing it and are at high risk for injuring your joints or muscles soon. When you feel that your muscles are gradually becoming stronger and bigger sans the pain, then you're doing it at the right intensity. No pain and no gains whatsoever...that's too light.

## Body Weight

While your ultimate goal is to be shredded and light through calisthenics, you may need to lose some pounds first by doing some cardio and eating better. Here's why you may need to do that.

Calisthenics is all about bodyweight. If you haven't done any regular exercise or fitness program, chances are you're not yet strong enough to support and move your bodyweight when executing the many different exercises and street workout routines. So you have the double whammy of excess weight and insufficient strength. You'll need to be able to reduce the gap between the two, at least just enough for you to be able to do the basic movements and routines well.

I have found that the safest way to lose excess weight in preparation for more intense fitness routines is by eating smart and doing regular aerobic exercises. Let's talk about eating smart first.

Eating smart for fat loss isn't rocket science. You simply make smarter food choices by eating more whole and un-processed foods and eating less. That's it. For example, by simply cutting out sugary processed foods like donuts and sweet pastries from your daily diet and replacing them with more fruits, veggies, or lean protein, you can already improve your body's chances of losing fat. One way to kick start this is to avoid any carbohydrates for the 1st week and stick to healthy, low-fat sources of protein. By depleting your body's carbs and glycogen stores for one week, you'll help your body use more body fat for its daily needs. Then after one week, start eating normally but healthier.

Of course, all the smart eating in the world won't do much if you don't burn more calories than what you normally eat. For beginners, the best way is to start by doing regular aerobic exercise – and I don't mean you should slip into those leotard tights and dance like Richard Simmons. You can start with brisk walking daily for at least 30 minutes and make sure you're exercise intensity is moderate. Once it becomes light to you, increase your pace and gradually transition into running.

Another fun way of doing aerobic exercise is riding your bike. As with brisk walking, ensure you're exercising at moderate intensity. If you you're intensity is low, you can compensate by lengthening your exercise session accordingly.

## Warming Up and Stretching

Whether its calisthenics or aerobics, you should warm up

the particular muscles that will be involved prior to working out. Why? It ensures that your muscles are flexible and loose enough to handle the good stress of your workout routine.

Regarding stretching, it's best to go for dynamic stretching rather than static. Dynamic stretching involves movement while dynamic stretching involves holding a stretched position for a fixed period of time. Walking, and mimicking the movements of the workout you'll do are forms of dynamic stretching and is a lot gentler on stiff and cold muscles compared to static stretching, which forces your cold muscles to stretch immediately. Studies have reported that static stretching actually increases your risk for injuries if done prior to working out. As such, it's best that you do dynamic stretches prior to the workout and static stretches afterwards.

*Andrew Creager*

# Chapter 12

# Street Workouts for Absolute Beginners

If you're completely new to strength training exercises and are not overweight to begin with, it's best to start working out your body as a whole before going into muscle group-specific training. Why? It's because to effectively train your individual muscle groups, you'll need to first develop a good and balanced overall strength level. Imagine if you start working out your chest and neglect your back – you'll only succeed at creating a strength imbalance between your front and back, which increases your risks for injuries. By doing full-body workouts at the beginning, you're able to achieve good overall strength and balance that's necessary for effectively training individual muscle groups later on.

## Beginners' Street Workout #1

This routine is gender-neutral, i.e., beneficial for both men and women.  The beauty of this routine is that it allows you to execute movements even if you're not yet strong enough to support your own body weight with the help of resistance bands.  Here's the routine:

1.     Begin with 5 reps of resistance band-assisted chin-ups. If you find that you can't just pull yourself up with your own strength, use a resistance band to assist in pulling your self up.  Tie a resistance band of sufficient tension to the bar you'll be pulling yourself up from.  Insert a foot into the handle and step on it until it stretches to the ground.  Pull yourself up and allow the resistance band to "push" you from your foot to help you complete the pull-ups.  If you still find it quite difficult, replace the band with one of higher tension.

2.     If you're still unable to do the resistance band-assisted pull-ups, you can replace it with negative pull-ups.  To execute a negative pull-up, you hold the bar above you with both hands and propel yourself into a pulled-up position by jumping.  From that position, gradually lower yourself to the ground.  The emphasis is on the negative phase of the pull-up's movement, which is the descent, by resisting the

movement down. Do 5 reps at first and gradually increase as you become stronger.

3.    Next exercise is resistance band-assisted dips. This is basically the normal dip exercise using a dipping bar but since you're still a beginner, you can tie a resistance band on both bars on which you can rest or hook both your feet on top to give you an extra push as you dip and come up. Do five reps of this and gradually increase as your strength does.

4.    If you're not yet strong enough for resistance band-assisted dips, you can do the simple bench dip. Sit on the edge of a sturdy bench, support your weight by planting your palms strongly on both your sides on the bench and move your butt off the bench. Lower your body as far as you can before rising back up to complete one rep. You push of with your arms to rise back up and use your legs to provide just enough assistance to your triceps to complete the movements.

5.    The next movement is the knee-pushup. This is an easier variant of the standard pushups, where instead of planking your whole body straight from the toes to the

arms, you'll be planking from the knees instead. The shorter plank distance makes it easier for you as a beginner to execute the movement and do so properly until you become strong enough to do the regular standard pushup. Do 5 repetitions and gradually increase as you become stronger.

6. Lastly, do 5 reps of regular bodyweight squats. Stand straight, feet shoulder-width apart (or wider if it's uncomfortable or keeps you from executing the movement properly) and put your hands behind your head. Lower your body just until your hamstrings are parallel to the floor before rising up to your original position. Make sure your knees never go past your toes to minimize unnecessary strain on your knees.

Do 3 cycles of this routine 3 to 4 times per week until you become strong enough to advance to intermediate level workouts.

## Beginners' Street Workout #2

In this beginner's street workout routine, you'll do 5 exercises that are great for helping you transition into harder and more challenging street workouts.

1.    Australian pull-ups:  position yourself under a low-lying bar from which you can pull yourself up from a lying position.  Lie under the bar, with the bar at around your chest area.  Reach for the bar with both hands about shoulder-width apart, straighten your whole body, and pull yourself up until your body touches the bar before lowering down.  Do 5 reps.

2.    Lying Knee-Tucks:  While lying straight on the ground, pull your knees toward your torso and return to starting position.  Do 5 reps.

3.    Lunges:  Start with your right leg.  Stand straight, put your right foot about a foot and a half in front of you and your left foot about the same distance behind you.  Lower your body until your right thigh is parallel to the floor then bring yourself up.  Do 5 reps of this before switching to the other leg for another 5 reps.

4.    Knee-Pushups:  Same as workout #1 earlier, plank yourself from the knees instead of your feet and do 5 pushups.

Do 5 sets or cycles of this routine 3 to 4 times weekly until you develop enough strength to do the harder workouts.

# Chapter 13
# Intermediate Level Street Workouts

Once you've gotten the hang of the beginner's level street workout routines, it's time to up the ante. Hold your horses – we're not yet talking of the hardcore stuff but an in-between level that will be help you transition well into the big leagues of calisthenics street workouts.

## Intermediate Street Workout Routine #1

This is the simpler routine between the 2 in this chapter. Complete 3 sets or cycles of this routine with 90 second rest periods in between 3 times per week.

1.    Static Chin-ups: To do this, jump and assume the peak or top position of a standard bar chin up and hold the position for 5 seconds before lowering yourself back to original position. Do 8 reps per set or cycle.

2.    Elevated Pushups:    This is a good halfway point between the real deal and your initial knee-pushups.  You execute standard pushups – planked from the feet instead of from the knees – but instead of pushing yourself from the floor, push yourself against a sturdy bench or elevated platform.  Do 10 reps of this.

3.    Leg Raises:    Lie straight on the floor or on a bench (with your butt near the end of the bench), straighten your legs and raise them until they're perpendicular to the floor or straight up before lowering to the starting position.  Do 10 reps.

4.    Angled Bar Rows:    Look for a bar in the playground that's just about chest height.    Under the bar, form a straight line at a 45-degree angle from the floor, holding on to the bar to help you hold that pose.  At this point, the bar should be right above crotch area and your feet 1 to 2 feet in front of the bar.  Execute the movement by pulling yourself up until your body touches the bar, keeping your body straight and your feet planted.  Do 15 reps.

5.    Bench Dips:    Sit on the edge of a sturdy bench or bar and support yourself with your hands on it.    Lower your

body and straighten your legs. Push yourself up before lowering down. Do 10 reps.

6.    Bodyweight Squats:   Stand straight, feet shoulder width apart and arms straight in front of you. Lower your body until your thighs are parallel to the floor – keeping your knees from going past your toes – before standing back up. Do 20 reps.

## Intermediate Street Workout Routine #2

This is the harder of the 2 intermediate level workouts. Do 5 sets or cycles of this routine with 90 seconds of rest between each cycle for 3 times weekly.

1.    Standard Pull-ups:  Do 10 repetitions.

2.    Standard Pushups:  Do 20 repetitions.

3.    Hanging Leg Raises:  Do 15 repetitions.

4.    Angled Bar Rows:  Do 10 repetitions.

5.    Bar Dips:  Do 10 repetitions.

6.    Jumping Squats:  Do 20 repetitions.

*Andrew Creager*

# Chapter 14

# Leg Day

One of the most feared aspects about working out is leg day. It rings true to everyone who looks back on when they first started working out, but I assure you that you will come to love it. The importance of leg day comes from the fact that you need a strong base. When your base is strong, you're going to be able to build off of that foundation. As you continue to work on your legs, you'll notice how much strength you truly possess in your thighs and calves. Here are four exercises that I strongly recommend for your maximum performance when it comes to building muscle in your legs.

## Squats:

Squats are an incredible and vital part of your workout. It's a workout that you should fit in no matter the amount of time you have to spend at the gym. Squats do so much for your body and really build your thighs.

To do a squat, start in a standing position with your hands by your sides. As you move your arms upward, bend at the knees and hold that position. Keep your back as straight as possible as you go into the squatting position. Then moving your arms back to your sides, stand. Take it slow, make sure that your back is straight, and be sure to push up from your butt. Another thing to check for is that your knees do not bend over your toes. Think of your squats as sitting down, not as crouching.

## Calf Raises:

This exercise is easy to perform but will really work the calves. Stand in front of a wall at a distance and lean against it with both hands at shoulder height. Then raise your feet so that all of your weight goes onto your toe area. Repeat the exercise and make sure that your body is straight at all times. Now wrap your left foot behind your right knee and do the lift again, swapping position to exercise the other side.

## Thigh Exercises

It's important to exercise your thigh area because this is an area which can get flabby. With today's lifestyles, I found that I was sitting down far too much of the time and this exercise helps you to address that. Side lunges allow you to exercise one side at a time. Stand with your legs together. Move your right leg away from your left leg forward and slightly to the side and as it touches the ground lunge down so that the knee is bent and then back up to the standing position. You should feel the stretch in the upper leg area as you put your weight on the bent knee. When you have finished exercising that leg, use your other leg and perform the same exercise. You will get into a rhythm with these and doing them to music is also great fun.

## Inner Thigh Area

These exercises will help to tame your inner thigh area. Lateral Leg lifts are great for this. Stand with your legs apart, place your hands on your hips and raise your left leg to the side and back again. Do this continually for ten repetitions and then change legs.

Standing leg circles are another exercise which is fairly easy to do, but which stretches the leg and works the muscles in the inner thigh. Stand with feet together, move your right leg up and forward and make circling motions with the whole leg ten times before replacing the leg onto the exercise mat. Now do the same with the other leg. This will also work for the hip area and is very good for mobility.

## Clamshell exercises

These are great for working out your legs. Lie on your side on the mat but make sure that your legs are bent, rather than straight. This is important, as your legs should stay bent throughout the exercise. Lift the top leg and then put it back to just above the lower leg but not touching it. Repeat this 10 times, lifting as far as you can and taking the exercise slowly so that it gets a chance to work the muscles. You will feel this one, but the weight of the movement is what is working the leg muscles.

Between exercises you can use walk steps that simply relax the muscles a little if you feel too much pull. Using walk steps on the spot helps you to get ready for the next exercise and is always a good way to stop cramps from developing in your legs and hips. The most important thing when exercising parts of you that haven't been exercised in a while is to drink water to stop cramping from happening, as this hydrates the body.

*Andrew Creager*

# Chapter 15
# Core

For many people, the area of their body that they want to get toned the fastest is their core. Everyone wants a flat stomach, or a six-pack for that matter. If you're looking for a tummy that is tight and straight, I've got another four exercises that are going to radically change your stomach and tighten up that core. Remember, core is important. It will influence everything you do and should therefore be taken extremely seriously.

**The Planks:**

Planks are simply lying on your stomach and then pushing up with your elbows and the tips of your toes, turning your body into a plank. You hold this pose for thirty to sixty seconds per exercise. This might sound like nothing, but just wait until around ten seconds into it before you start saying otherwise. The great thing about planks is that there are multiple variations, including: Side planks, where you do a plank but propping yourself up on your side with an elbow and the side of your foot. Mountain climbers: where you bring your knees up to your chest one at a time while you continue to hold the pose. Crawlers: Instead of bringing your knees up to your chest, bring them up from the side. All of these will radically transform your core.

## Reverse Crunches:

Lie on your back and look up at the ceiling for this exercise. Now, I want you to keep your legs straight while bringing your toes up as high as you can, all the way until your knees are just inches from your chest. Lift up your pelvis as much as you can so that it feels like you're folding in. Now, I want you to slowly lower your legs back to their resting point— slowly! Don't just drop your legs. You'll feel the burn as you're doing it. This really works your core at its base.

## Elbow Crunches:

This is a great workout for your butt and abs. Lie down on your exercise mat and facing downwards rest your weight onto your elbows. Flex one of your legs and give it a lift because this really works the core. You need to really punch upward with your heel, rather than your toe and pull in the abs area of the body. You may find on your initial tries that you sink toward the floor, but keep those arms straight and your spine straight.

**The Plank:**

Move from the last position so that your legs are stretched out behind you and you are taking the weight of your body on your hands. In this case, the reason this is called the plank is because of the straightness of the body. Move one leg so that the knee is bent and the foot is placed against the straight leg into a V. For this exercise you move the V down and then up again keeping your leg in that same position. Repeat this ten times and then switch sides. This is a very good exercise for mobility of the hips and will help keep the butt trim.

**Heel Touches:**

For this exercise, lie on your back and look at the ceiling. Bring your feet up so that your knees are pointed up toward the ceiling. Now as you lie on the floor, reach around and touch the heel of your foot. It will be: right hand touches right heel and left hand touches left heel. That will equal one rep. Ensure you don't just shrug down, but actually reach while remaining on your back. Do this until exhaustion for the maximum reward.

If you can master these four workouts on your core day for the next six weeks, you're going to see dramatic results in your core strength and your weight. If you're looking to define your core, these exercises are all about toning and sculpting as well. With the right nutrition, dedication, and intensity, you'll have that core you always wanted in no time.

To learn more about core exercises, go check out bar brothers YouTube channel. They have 20+ exercises on there; I am just getting your feet wet. When choosing a YouTube video to work with, choose one where the participant has the same style of body as you do and is of the same sex because women's exercises may vary a little from the male variety.

# Chapter 16

# Chest

Most men really want a well-defined chest and women want the opposite. Most women are afraid that working out their chest will actually make their breasts smaller. This is not the case at all. In fact, it's the opposite. By building up the muscle in your chest, you will have a more pronounced and defined chest, regardless of your gender and everyone wants that. So let me give you some exercises that will really help define your chest and give you what it is you want most out of your chest workout: results.

## Pushups:

Pushups are amazing because there is so much you can do with them and you really don't need equipment to do these. After each exercise, be sure to take a break of about 30 seconds and then move onto the next version of the push up. The push up position is where you are on your knees and lean forward so that your hands are on the mat in front of you but wide enough to take your weight. Now move your legs back so that you are balancing the legs on your toes. Lift the left leg. Lower the body until your arms bend and then pull up, keeping the one leg off the floor. Work 6 repetitions and then change sides. When you have finished, straighten the arms and sit up taking deep breaths to let your body catch up. Your body should always be in a straight line when you perform this exercise and your arms bent to the side at shoulder level.

Next kneel and then get back into the lying down position, but be careful to stretch the legs out behind you and place your arms so that the bend and the arms are parallel with your shoulder. It's more to the side than in front of you. Keeping your body in that plank position with your spine straight, lift your weight up and then back down again. This is strenuous exercise so take it slowly at first and don't try too many repetitions if you feel strained. Your breathing is important during the exercise and you will need to breathe in deeply and breathe out equally intensely.

You will find that these exercises are great for the core area and particularly the chest and abs. You may find yourself bending a little at first but be conscious of the straightness needed and correct your position. When you have learned to do these two exercises easily, then time yourself instead of counting. Give yourself up to 15 minutes and 20 max.

**The Corkscrew :**

Taking the same stance as in the last exercise, move your right arm position so that an angle is created, your left hand at waist level and your right arm a little above your head. This corkscrew motion used during pushups really does work the muscles in your chest and your abs. Take it a little slow to start off with. With your hands correctly placed, start to do your pushups. Repeat 5 times and then change sides.

**Narrow Pushups:**

In this exercise, take the normal push up stance, but place your hands close to your body at just above waist height. It will take some pushing but push your body upward keeping your spine straight. Let the body down again. This exercise is high intensity and uses the body weight to really make your muscles work hard.

# Chapter 17

# Back

The back is an easy place to really forget or relegate as useless when you're working out. After all, how often do you really use your back? The answer is: always. Your back is vital for you to look your best. When you workout your shoulders, your chest, and your core, all those muscles are getting larger, pulling on ligaments and bones as they get tighter and stronger. So, if you don't workout your back, you start to slouch. By working out your back, you're going to really see a change in overall definition because your posture is getting better and stronger for you. Here are some exercises for your back that are really going to help in getting the rest of your body to peak condition.

## Lower Back Area

This exercise actually targets the lower back area. Lie face down and stretch your arms as far up as you can above your head. Press your hands onto the floor and, trying to keep your back as straight and stretched as possible, lift your thighs. This exercise should be repeated several times, but work up to doing as many as ten because, once again, you won't be used to using these muscles, so a few at a time, increasing as you get more experienced is better than racing at it.

## Exercise 2 – Lower back

You need to be in the same position so this exercise ideally follows the last exercise. This time press down on the floor with your toes and lift your body from the waist upward keeping your arms outstretched, rather than using them to push you.

# Chapter 18
# Shoulders

With shoulders, I want your mantra to be: have excellent form. Shoulder injuries are easy to acquire, but also easy to avoid. Remember to have good form and to take your workouts in a timely and controlled fashion. No jerking and flailing. Got it? Now, the great thing about shoulders is that it'll revolutionize the way clothing hangs on you. Great shoulders provide great silhouettes and even better figure for your upper body. So here's how you can really get the most out of your shoulder workout.

## Side Delts

These are exercises that are used to help you to strengthen up your shoulders and unlike other exercises, which use equipment, this exercise uses your own body weight and that's a lot easier to do in your own time and space without having to visit a gym. This exercise using the standard plank position, where your body forms a straight plank on the carpet, but you lean your weight upon your elbows. You are effectively going to roll to one side, keeping the weight of the body on that one elbow that touches the mat. Move the arm that is not supporting you away from your body so that it gives full stretch to the muscles. This is quite a strenuous exercise so try two repetitions with each side of the body at first. If you feel that your shoulders need a bit more work, you can increase this later.

## Shoulder Flexibility

Perhaps you don't want to build up the muscle on your arms and shoulders but just want to add to the flexibility of the shoulder joint. This is quite possible since these can get stiff even from carrying too much shopping. The best exercise for this is shoulder rolls and rotating the arms. If you stand with your legs slightly apart, to give you a good comfortable base, start to move your arms to the front and around reaching as far as you can with each movement. Then rotate in the opposite direction.

Body weight is useful for exercise, and for this exercise, you need to place yourself lying face downward on the mat. Now, make a plank by balancing on the toe area of your food and pulling your upper torso off the mat with your arms.

To strengthen the shoulders, you need to balance on one hand at a time, rotating the other arm until it has moved full circle. Place it back onto the mat and repeat. Then change sides because this will help to give the shoulders a lot of flexibility.

The shoulders are a hard area of the body to really get an amazing workout and it's also really easy to injure yourself if you're not careful with the weight of the body and how you are positioned. But, if you're looking for some exercises to get a really solid, rounded workout, try some of these. Really commit to sculpting and building your shoulders over the next several weeks when it comes to be your shoulder day.

*Andrew Creager*

# Chapter 19

# Arms

Finally, we come to the last body part that we're going to work out and that's the arms. Generally, I would suggest that you break up your arms between biceps and triceps so that you're not working both in the same day. However, when it comes to arms, it is vital that you give them a strong, solid workout. Every man wants big arms and every woman wants toned arms, both are excellent goals and I'm going to explain with both areas why you should invest heavily in them. However, in the end, I'm going to discuss forearms, because when I was starting training, I was really curious about how to build my forearms as well as my biceps and triceps. So, let's get started with this.

**Biceps:**

You may not feel that these can be exercised without

weights, but you would be wrong. Stand with your feet slightly apart so that you are comfortable and steady. Stretch your arms out to the side and rotate them in a very small rotation, wiggling your fingertips at the same time. The wiggling motion is great because it's getting your arm muscles into movement and without even knowing it, you are already starting your exercise routine. Try to avoid lifting your shoulders because the movement should be more fluid. You can keep doing this exercise for a full five minutes followed by placing your palms in an upward direction. Now push the arms up and down to the side of you. They don't need to travel a lot of distance, but you need consistent pushes that will work all the small muscle groups in turn.

## Triceps:

For this area of the arm, stay in the same position but fold your arms upward. Keeping your arm at this angle, move it in a downward motion and then back to the original position. Try not to move the shoulders. This is all about the triceps and you should begin to feel them pull. This is great exercise for keeping your arms in tiptop condition.

## Forearms:

For the forearm area a whole arm workout does the trick so do the exercises as shown above but this time add another. With your arms out to the side and bent at a right angle, make a small movement upward and then a full movement upward until the arm is fully stretched. Repeat this up to ten times. It works on the groups of muscles in the forearms as well as working on triceps and biceps and is a great warming up exercise that will energize you.

When it comes to arms, a lot of people want to really define their progress by how big or how toned their arms are. That is fine. Just remember that all progress is about form and consistency. While arm workouts might seem repetitive and boring, that's because they are. There are variations to give you some new flavor and some new chances to hit the muscles from different angles, but that's about it. As you progress through training, you're going to find different, unique exercises for the arms that look great. Go ahead and try them, incorporate them and mix them up. Whatever works for you. Just keep working out!

*Andrew Creager*

# Chapter 20
# Planning Your Workout Regimen

Now that you have made it this far into the book, you have a pretty good idea of what you should and should not do. You know that you will need to properly plan your workout routine rather than just jumping into it.

After you have visited your physician and decided what types of exercises are safe for you to do, you can now successfully plan your week according to the order of exercises that works best for you. When planning your workout, it is important that you keep the target area of every exercise in mind. You do not want to focus on the same target area two days in a row so it is important to plan carefully.

The order in which you target your muscles is completely up to you. Just keep in mind that you do not want to over exert important groups.

## Taking Time for Cardio

If one of your main objectives is to lose weight and tone muscle, you will not want to miss out on the extraordinary benefits of a cardio workout. Performing a cardio workout before your typical exercise session can help you burn fat and build muscle faster than you would with lifting weights alone.

Over time, you may advance to using weights in your cardio workout, but it is not recommended for you to use weights at first. This is because cardio workouts cause you to move in ways that your body is not expecting. If it does not have the proper strength to support the weight you are carrying, along with a free weight, you could cause a serious muscle strain, sprain, or even tear. The last thing you want to do is cause yourself serious injury right out of the gate so you should take it slow.

## Beginning Cardio

While you may feel the urge to jump right into a rigorous cardio workout and start melting away fat, it is best to start with low impact cardio workouts that provide exercise in short, steady bursts. This will allow you to slowly adjust to the impact that your body will experience from high impact exercise.

After you have become comfortable with the movements in a beginners cardio routine, you can work your way up to intermediate and then advanced. It is important that you do not push yourself too fast into the skill.

## Ways to Build Up for Cardio

Many view cardio as a snooze fest, necessary evil, and mostly like some impossible task. But it is not. Its positive effects are there in our faces every day. Many people actually are unable to put a finger on effective cardio.

Gone are the times when jogging around town or an hour in the park could help make you fit. A successful cardio routine however ensures that you get and remain fit. Here are some ways that can help with that.

-Plan accordingly. Know what you are doing and plan according to that, say go to two to three sessions of workout that progressively get harder as you work more. If you are able to handle more, it indicates that you are getting better at it and progressing.

-Timing. This is important for people who usually end up skipping their cardio. It is advised that you usually do it just before hitting the gym or on days off. Just do not skip.

-Focus. Keep your hands empty and do one thing at a time.

-Warm up. This will increase mobility and help avoid any injury as such. Don't overlook doing a warm-up before cardio.

-Avoid steady pace cardio. Apply varying degrees of pace to your cardio workout. This will even help boost metabolism.

-Sprint. Incorporate it into the workout.

-Mix in exercises. This is just to shuffle up the routine and avoid making it boring. Throw in a couple of bodyweight exercises and mix them up a little.

-Keep yourself motivated. That little voice in the back of your head telling you to break and slow down, don't listen.

-Cool down. As said previously, this is very important. It speeds up the recovery process.

-Keep track of your workout. Make a note of weight lifted or the tempo maintained. This will help you be aware of your body's capabilities and how far can you push it.

-Final and foremost is consistency. Just doing cardio every once in a little while will not help. It is imperative that one maintains consistency.

The results will show later of doing cardio consistently for an extended period of time. And you can be assured that they won't disappoint.

*Andrew Creager*

# Chapter 21

# Cardio Workouts and Their effectiveness

When coupled with proper weight training, a cardio workout is bound to give you the ideal body shape and weight loss.

Get over the fear of boredom from cardio and try out these workout routines that will give you results that you will love.

## The Stairmaster

The stair climbing machine is bound to stimulate the cardio workout. It targets the glutes and helps produce an adequate amount of sweat. It's great for fat loss. The idea is to maintain a certain amount of intensity and avoid slacking off on it. It's not like a typical treadmill.

Do a thirty to twenty minute workout on it for up to two or

three times a week. It can be used both for High-intensity interval training (HIIT) and the low-intensity steady-state cardio (LISS). Any of the styles deliver great results.

An effective method is to try alternate styles, which can help focus on the glutes and thighs, as well as the rest of the body. Push your limits and challenge yourself. That is the key.

## Pyrometrics

This is challenging, yet highly interesting. This gets the heartbeat pumping and requires intense focus. It's basically like doing the jumping jacks, hence are convenient and easily adaptable. Even people with less flexibility can attempt this.

Do as many as you can in twenty seconds, then break for the same time. Go up a notch to thirty, then rest. Progress higher each time and repeat.

Doing up to three and four cycles can account for quick, effective cardio.

## Running

This is pretty basic. A run in the park or a hop on the treadmill can actually contribute to a good cardio workout. Apart from the physical aspect, it also helps with mental health. Stress relief is one of its healthy by-products. For busy people, it may be exactly what they need and provide them with relaxation.

Put in yourheadphones, shut out the world, and go for a run. This will not only ease stress but also burn fat. Incorporate it into the workout.

Do small fifteen to ten seconds sprints then slow to a walk and rest. Go up to ten to twelve rounds and feel the difference in yourself.

## Jumping Rope

One can either do this stand alone or make it a part of the routine. It's effective when there is less time and one might need to work up a quick sweat. You can use a routine of your choice, mixing it up with different speeds and time rests. It can be done anywhere and only requires a rope.

Do fifty to one hundred jumps in between exercises or maybe for an interval of thirty to sixty seconds.

It is great for keeping the heart rate up and making a good interesting workout routine.

These are the workouts that can lead to fast burning of fat and leave you with a lean, solid shape.

Apart from these there are other effective workouts for cardio as well. Crunches, bicycling, bodyweight squats, pull-ups, ab rolls, and leg raises among others.

These workouts may be intense; hence it is important that one focuses on doing a single routine each week and then progress to two or three as the body gets conditioned to it. The trick is to rest little and continue with it in one go. Break just long enough to control the heartbeat and then move on.

Other than that there are workouts for cardio that can easily be done at home and need no equipment.

There are ways to do a lower or upper body workout combined with other exercises at home. Take breaks, stretch, and cool down properly. Remember to push yourself and take the challenge head on.

These workouts include:

Up & Over Steps-High Knee Pulls

Butt Kicker Drops-Jumping Jack Squat

Plank Jack along with Knee Countdown Squats

Toe Touch Jacks-Center Hop Pushes

Up & Out Jacks-Lateral Hops and Knee

Alternating Lunge and Twist

Lat Pull-down and Standing Row

Time yourself for forty-five to sixty seconds for each routine with fifteen seconds break.

Everything is easier these days and can be easily done at home, even if you have no equipment. At home exercises are convenient for people with hectic busy lives and little spare time. Try to do these cardio workouts and feel the difference in yourself.

## Make Cardio More Effective

-Pick the right machines. For example, ellipticals with levers will make for a better workout as the movement of arms back and forth will help level blood flow and activate muscles.

-Grip the frame of the machine. That is bound to easy up the workout.

-Stay focused on burning up the calories instead of giving too much attention to the numbers. Forget numbers and push yourself hard.

-Pay attention to the response of the body to a particular exercise. Listen to the body and figure out how it feels after you have finished.

Cardio is important and should be a part of your exercise regime. Make it fun with the help of music, partners, and different workout routines every day, and you will find yourself living a healthy, better life with increased mobility, agility, and good shape.

# Chapter 22
# Supplements

With the wide variety of supplements available at health food stores and online, it can be difficult to determine what you should and should not use in conjunction with your workout. As I stated in the introduction to this book, I will only be recommending two supplements for your workout routine, multi-vitamins and creatine.

While adding more vitamins to your workout may seem like it would help you to increase your exercise potential, the truth is they can hold you back and many of them are toxic to your body.

## Side Effects of Other Vitamins

Most vitamins that are geared toward exercise contain ingredients that have not been proven safe by the FDA, or any other health agency. These vitamins cause a large percentage of hospitalizations each year. Some can lead to stroke; others can lead to heart attack and even death. Because of the uncertainty and the various health reports, I will not be recommending them, nor do I condone the use of these supplements.

## The Purpose of a Multi-Vitamin

Adding a multi-vitamin to your daily regimen can greatly increase your health in many ways. Scientists claim that we must take in a certain amount of each vitamin in order to remain healthy. The problem is that no one really has time to monitor how much of each vitamin he or she are taking in, or the stomach capacity to eat enough of each food group to reach the daily recommended value. A multi-vitamin can dramatically increase your chances of hitting the target for each and every recommended vitamin.

## Creatine

In the introduction to this book, I mentioned a substance called creatine. Many people have heard the word, but they don't know the true reason for taking it during a workout regimen. By understanding its reaction with the body, you can easily determine the importance of the nutrient and why you should take it on a regular basis.

Creatine is a component that is present in all living things. It is stored in the muscles and is used to fuel them, and help them contract when needed. Without enough of this essential muscular component, your muscles cannot function at their peak, leaving you weak and prone to injury and accidents.

Understanding how these vitamins can help you to increase your maximum performance will dramatically help you to build muscle, stay healthy, and prevent accidents in the gym or in other exercise settings.

Creatine has been through generations of trials to prove the safety of the product. However, the product safety is not the main concern you should have when purchasing it. Always make sure to purchase from a reputable brand that has been tested by an independent laboratory. This ensures that you will be buying a quality product that has been proven safe in its current form, and that it meets the minimum requirements to do what it claims.

## Not All Supplements Are Made the Same

Just because a supplement claims to be safe and contains what is considered safe ingredients, there are always some catches. This is why I recommend purchasing only quality tested products.

Unlike prescription medications, supplements are not required to put every ingredient on the label. They are also not required to complete the same rigorous testing that prescription products must go through in order to be approved for sale.

# Chapter 23
# Diet

Changing your diet is something that should be done gradually. This is because your body needs to adjust slowly and making drastic changes in your life can cause a lot of difficulty when it comes to sticking with the change. The objective is to create a permanent lifestyle and build habits that last for years, not simply change a few things temporarily.

Developing a healthier lifestyle will make you feel more refreshed and energized for your workout, as well as provide more energy for your daily activities. You will notice over a very short period of time that simple changes in your diet and avoiding junk food will provide you with a dramatic boost in energy.

## Snacking – Negative Calorie Foods

You will be amazed to find out that there is a concept called negative calorie foods. These foods make the perfect snack for any time of the day, especially when you are on a diet.

So what is a negative calorie food? A negative calorie food is an indulgence that burns more calories chewing and digesting it than it actually contains. While this is not the typical name for these foods, you are very familiar with them. These foods are fruits and vegetables that do not contain starch.

Negative calorie foods should always be eaten in their raw form. This ensures that they provide nutrition, digest in a manner that makes them a negative calorie food, and that they are not chemically changed.

Examples of negative calorie foods are carrots, celery, broccoli, bell peppers, and any other vegetable that does not contain starch.

## Balancing Your Diet

Everyone talks about balancing your diet, but what does

that really mean? Throwing a food pyramid at you and saying eat this, that, and the other is not the answer. There are so many variations of the food pyramid and no one is certain which one to follow. Even the FDA changes the food pyramid on a whim when a new scientific study comes out. With all of this information being thrown at you, how can you truly balance your diet?

## Your Caloric Intake

Your caloric intake should be between 1,200 and 1,500 calories per day, depending on your level of activity. You should never follow a diet that is considered low calorie and you should avoid any diet that recommends that you eat less than 1,200 calories per day. Keep in mind that it takes at least 800 calories per day just to keep your brain functioning at full capacity.

It depends on your specific activities and the recommendation of your personal trainer and physician. While your personal trainer and physician can give you advice, the only way that you can determine exactly what your dietary needs are is to consult a nutritionist. However, I will give you some generalized advice based on medically accepted standards.

Your diet should be composed of three basic nutrients, carbohydrates, proteins and fats. These nutrients are the type of calories that your body needs to create energy and develop a healthier lifestyle.

## Carbohydrates

Healthy carbohydrates should make up between 50 or 60 percent of your daily calories. This is because healthy carbohydrates are turned directly into glucose to fuel the body. This is energy that can be used immediately or can be transformed into glycogen and used as energy stores. Glycogen is stored in your liver and in your muscles. You should not allow your diet to consist of bad carbohydrates or more than 60 percent of your daily intake. This is because excess glycogen cannot be stored. Once you have reached your daily storage allotment, your body begins turning the extra carbohydrates into fat.

There are two basic types of carbohydrates, healthy carbs and unhealthy carbs. Healthy carbohydrates act slower in the body. They also have a slower and less dramatic effect on your blood sugar. The majority of your daily carbohydrate allotment should come from this type of carb.

Unhealthy carbohydrates are found in foods that are commonly referred to as junk food. Cookies, soda, artificially sweetened drinks, and candy do not last long in the body. However, they raise your blood sugar extremely fast and drop it just as rapidly. Also, they do not keep you full as long as healthy carbohydrates do, so they can cause a vicious eating cycle resulting in weight gain.

## Proteins

Proteins should comprise between 12 to 20 percent of your daily caloric intake. Protein is necessary in order for your body to create energy and develop muscle. Protein can be stored in large amounts in the body and is used to fuel muscles during routine activities and your exercise program.

Protein can affect blood sugar, but it does not do so in a dramatic manner. It can also take most proteins between 2 to 4 hours to affect your blood sugar levels. However, even if you have a health condition that requires you to monitor your blood sugar, you will not notice much of a rise, as it does not cause serious fluctuations.

## Fats

Fat is packed with calories, no matter what type of fat it is. Your daily diet should consist of no more than 30 percent of healthy fat. Fat helps create energy in the body and it is a necessary staple in your life. Fats have many different purposes in the body, but only 10 percent of the fat you ingest is turned into glucose.

Fat itself does not have an effect on blood sugar. However, when combined with carbohydrates, it can help reduce the rate that blood sugar increases. Fat also helps slow the rate of digestion so if your blood sugar does increase, the fat can cause your blood sugar to linger at a higher level for an extended period of time.

There are many different types of fats for you to come into contact with. Some fats are better for you than others, but in small amounts, fat can be a fairly healthy component when used correctly in your diet.

It is best to choose fats like mono-unsaturated fats or polyunsaturated fats. You can identify these fats easily because they are liquid at room temperature. You should avoid saturated fats, and trans-fats, which are solid, or hardened, at room temperature. This is because once they cool off in your body; they go back to the solid state that they started and begin damaging your arteries.

## Consulting a Nutritionist

As you can see, there are pretty wide gaps in the medical recommendations compiled through scientific study. This is because every person needs a different amount of each component. The only way to find the right balance between these three main components is to seek the advice of a professional nutritionist after you have developed your exercise plan.

A nutritionist can help you plan based on your personal limits and can help you create the exact mix of components your body needs to keep up with your current lifestyle.

*Andrew Creager*

# Chapter 24

# Proteins

Speaking of proteins, it is the stuff from which muscles are built. If you don't get enough of it, you won't enjoy a Greek god-looking ripped body. Why? Low body fat with poor muscle mass will only make you look like you haven't eaten for a year, which isn't sexy at all. But with enough muscle (no, I'm not talking Dwayne "The Rock" Johnson-like muscle mass but more like Ryan Reynolds), you'll look really good.

So how much protein will your body really need to gain enough muscle to look like a ripped Greek god?

While there are different estimates of just how much protein you really need for increasing muscle mass or maintaining it, the differences aren't that far off and are actually within a good enough ballpark figure. The range from which the ideal daily protein consumption for building muscle mass ranges from 0.8 to 1.5 grams of protein per pound of bodyweight. So how do you know where in between should be your daily target? Let's consider your current state of fitness and goals.

If you're a healthy average but sedentary adult with no form of regular exercise whatsoever and no plans of changing that, then your daily protein requirement is between 0.5 to 0.7 grams of protein per pound of body weight. If you are somewhat active (i.e., have some regular form of exercise or would like to significantly alter your body composition or body fat levels) then 0.8 to 1.0 grams of protein per pound of bodyweight may be ideal for you.

However, if you're trying to build serious amounts of muscle, i.e., bodybuilding, then you'll need more. If you're a female bodybuilder or are planning to be one, you'll need at least 1 gram of protein per pound of bodyweight up to 1.2 grams. If you're male, then your daily protein requirements would be up to 1.5 grams of protein per pound of bodyweight.

A good rule of thumb to go by if you're not sure is that

which most fitness experts have used for the longest time – 1.0 gram per pound of bodyweight.

## How Much?

To get an estimate of how much you'll need based on your fitness goals and current weight, simply multiply your bodyweight as of the moment by the recommended protein amount per pound of bodyweight. It's that easy!

However, it'll be a bit different if you're currently obese. If you merely used your bodyweight as the basis for your daily protein requirements, then you'll overshoot your target and may end up gaining more fat in the process. To avoid this, use your target or ideal body weight as your basis. So instead of multiplying by your current body weight, multiply it by your desired one instead.

Keeping your protein consumption within the ranges identified above should be enough to help you maximize your calisthenics muscle building efforts.

## Ideal Sources

The best source of protein is whole foods and the following

is a list of such foods from <u>theconsciouslife.com</u>:

| Food | Quantity | Protein |
|------|----------|---------|
| Atlantic Herring | 1 Fillet (143g) | 32.93 |
| Cuttlefish | 100g | 32.48 |
| Alaskan Salmon (Canned) | 100g | 30.7 |
| Octopus | 100g | 29.82 |
| Roasted Chicken Breast | 1/2 Breast (98g) | 29.2 |
| Roasted Turkey Breast | 100g | 28.71 |
| Tuna | 100g | 28.21 |
| Braised Bottom Round Beef | 3 Oz ( 85g) | 27.85 |
| Tilapia | 100g | 26.15 |
| Broiled, Boneless Pork Sirloin | 3 Oz (85g) | 25.94 |

| | | |
|---|---|---|
| Alaskan King Crab | 1 Leg (134g) | 25.93 |
| Clam | 100g | 25.55 |
| Braised Pork Ribs | 3 Oz (85g) | 24.7 |
| Blue Mussel | 100g | 23.8 |
| Sardine, Canned In Tomato Sauce | 3 Sardines (114g) | 23.78 |
| Broiled Top Sirloin, Beef | 3 Oz (85g) | 22.92 |
| Cooked Lamb | 3 Oz (85g) | 21.68 |
| Atlantic Mackerel | 1 Fillet (146g) | 20.99 |
| Scallop | 100g | 20.54 |
| Shrimp | 3 Oz (85g) | 19.36 |
| Roasted Duck | 100g | 18.99 |
| Squid | 100g | 17.94 |

| Roasted Chicken Thigh | 1 Thigh (62g) | 15.54 |
|---|---|---|
| Roasted Chicken Drumstick | 1Drumstick (52g) | 14.06 |
| Hardboiled Egg | 2 Eggs (100g) | 12.58 |

Although this isn't an exhaustive list of high-protein foods, this should be more than enough to help you plan your daily meals and maximize your muscle building efforts.

**Protein Powders**

There are times, regularly in fact, that getting all of your muscle building protein requirements from whole foods can be very difficult. For one, you'll need to eat quite a volume to do so. Second, there are times that it's simply inconvenient to prepare that much food. Here's where protein powders can come in handy.

Protein powders can help you fill in those protein gaps to ensure you're getting enough protein to build muscle. Many athletes replace a meal or two with protein shakes to ensure they get their protein fills for the day.

Taking a whey protein shake before and after your workouts is the best way to supplement your daily protein requirements. In particular, whey protein is the fastest acting one, which your muscles need immediately prior to and after each calisthenics street workout session. But don't over do it. Whole foods are still the best way to go and to the extent possible, limit your whey protein shakes to pre and post workouts.

*Andrew Creager*

# Chapter 25
# Hydration

Hydration is one of the cornerstones of weight loss, feeling better, and developing a healthy body. The human body is comprised of 60 percent water. As you exercise you lose water from your body through sweat and you begin to become dehydrated. Without proper water and electrolyte intake, you can easily become dehydrated to the point of being lethargic, weak, and unable to regenerate muscle effectively. It also deprives your organs of the necessary fluids they need to remain healthy, leaving you at risk for becoming ill or damaging your organs if dehydration becomes a chronic problem.

Studies have proven that large majorities of people who exercise are chronically dehydrated meaning that they are not doing their body any favors and are in fact risking their long-term health.

It is recommended that the average person drinks at least 64 ounces of water per day. This is a well-known fact because doctors drill it into our heads constantly. What they do not tell you is that for every hour of exercise you perform, you should take in an extra eight ounces of water. If you are not compensating properly for the water being lost, you are sentencing yourself to being one of the people who are exercising in a state of chronic dehydration.

## Drinking Water

Drinking water on a regular basis can help keep you hydrated. However, it cannot replace the minerals that are lost during routine exercise. Despite its ability to keep a person hydrated.

Many of these minerals are hard to keep balanced after exercise, even if you intentionally ingest them in large quantities after exercise. These minerals can be obtained by taking a multi-vitamin on a regular basis and by drinking specially formulated drinks that contain them in the proper quantities.

## Sports Drinks

While water is a great method of rehydration, sports drinks can help replace the electrolytes that you lose during exercise. As you sweat, you lose more than just water; you lose sodium, vitamins, and minerals as well. Sports drinks help to replace these lost chemicals that are vital to your body functioning at full capacity. Choosing a reputable sports drink or an electrolyte replacement powder that mixes well with filtered or bottled water can help replace what you lose during your workout.

*Andrew Creager*

# Chapter 26
# Ways to Make Exercise Fun for Everyone

Reaching the end, I would like to talk about ways where you can make exercise fun for everyone, including family and friends. When people usually hear exercise, they tend to shy away from it. Reasons for this can be lethargy or just because they find it boring.

Here are some ways in which you can engage everyone:

Fitness is usually associated with going to the gym. This does not necessarily have to be the case. There are fun alternatives that are just as healthy.

Go outside; familiarize your family and friends with outdoor activities. In today's day and age, children from age five and above are more engrossed in smartphones, tablets, and video games that they hardly tend to go outside.

This is one of the primary reasons why young teenagers display tendencies of obesity and are overweight. Their outdoor activities are almost negligible. Fitness problems such as restricted movement and RSI (repetitive strain injuries) arise because of being positioned in one angle.

Obviously when one is fixated on their phone or computer, they are not moving very much. To counter this, suggest exciting activities like hiking, trekking, biking, or even skating. All these are healthy and help a person stay active.

Instill the discipline of exercise in children from an early age. Take them to the gym if it allows and show them around. Most gyms allow children from age twelve and above, so if your child is of that age, don't leave them behind somewhere.

Show them weights and fun exercises that build their interest in keeping healthy and fit.

These habits if developed properly stay with kids for years to come.

If going on a holiday, whether with friends or family, chalk in some physical activities. Go for water sports, skiing, mountain climbing, or any such activities that help people maintain a healthy lifestyle and develop their interest in fitness.

You might also get to indulge in activities that you have never done before and might enjoy them. If the group of people around you is of an older age, try arranging strength training contests. Create a challenging situation where everyone has to lift strengths according to their body weights.

If it's possible in your family, keep it between that. It will be fun for them if the entire family can be engaged in such an activity. Keep it fair, giving each one weights that they can handle and push them to test their limits.

A family that works out together stays together. You can see that even among celebrities and athletes. David Beckham and his family, especially his oldest son are frequently photographed going together to SoulCycle sessions. That way the entire family can be seen looking great and fit.

When you are trying to engage a group of people in activities, try to cater to everyone's choice. Take turns picking activities. In this way, everyone will be interested and there will be more variety.

As said earlier, organize outdoor activities. Play games outside, not just your average Frisbee or hopscotch. Try to indulge in sports. Like football or badminton.

Host sporting events and involve the entire community or neighborhood. It could be a match of rugby, soccer, or baseball. It could be anything that involves running around and muscle flexibility.

Finally, this may seem funny. But if you can, get a dog or a pet. Studies have shown that people with dogs or cats walk around thirty percent more than people who have none.

Try and apply these ways to attract and engage more people to exercising, staying fit, and moving towards leading a healthy lifestyle.

# Chapter 27
# Yoga – The Exercise of Endurance

If you are looking for an exercise that tests your endurance, burns calories, and helps work those hard to reach muscles, yoga may be just what you are looking for. Yoga may seem like a graceful, girly form of exercise, but in truth, it is an exercise of strength, endurance, power, and stamina.

Many people laugh at yoga when they first see it. They are unsure of whether or not they will gain anything from it or they think that it is just some meditation and relaxation method. The truth is yoga is a hard-core exercise program that can bring even the strongest man to his knees if sustained long enough.

All yoga exercises rely on pure strength. Difficult poses are held for long durations of time, strengthening muscles faster and burning fat at astronomical rates.

Yoga is the fastest way to build your core muscles and develop stronger ligaments and tendons. While most men look at yoga as a women's exercise, they are extremely surprised to find out that it is a challenge, no matter what your exercise

When combined with weight lifting and cardio workouts, you will see an amazing response from your body. You will burn fat and gain muscle at a rate that you never thought possible.

## Take it Slow

It is important that you take it slow in order to prevent injury to your large muscle groups and prevent pulling or straining a tendon or muscle. Knowing your limitations will help you to ensure that you are able to avoid injury.

Learning yoga is not something that you will want to do on your own. Even if you do not plan to take classes long term, it is important that you take classes for a while to ensure that you develop the right form to ensure that you do not cause injury.

## Yoga Can Be Dangerous

While yoga is a very beneficial exercise program, it is a very dangerous exercise program. You use muscles to support your weight that most people are not familiar with using. You must be ready and willing to experience some form of pain during and after exercise after you start the program, because yoga will make muscles hurt that you did not even know existed.

While it is tempting, you will want to avoid any activity that involves standing on your head without some sort of neck support. There have been countless neck injuries caused by people doing yoga poses that involve standing on their head on a yoga mat and losing their balance. There is an extremely high risk of causing permanent damage, paralysis, or collapsing vertebra.

## Take the Proper Precautions

There are many different precautions that you should take before and during a yoga exercise program. You should always stretch your body out completely before you begin a session. Make sure that you are able to properly preform an exercise under supervision before you decide to do it alone at home.

Just like any other exercise, you will want to properly stretch and warm up before completing a yoga exercise program. Failing to stretch properly for a yoga session can be more dangerous than failing to stretch for a standard exercise. This is because during yoga, you are required to hold extremely difficult poses for a long duration of time.

## Adjusting Your Yoga Workout to Suit Your Needs

When you are beginning a yoga exercise program, you should ensure that it is customized to your personal needs. It is easy to overdo yoga because even though it is a very stressful exercise for your muscles, it is also a very relaxing form of exercise. Because of this, you can easily over work your muscles and cause excessive soreness.

In order to determine your endurance level, you should start with a beginner's class at a local gym and learn simple stretches and poses to start with. Once you have mastered simple poses, you can slowly increase your knowledge of yoga and increase the number of poses that you can complete during a standard session. You may want to alternate poses each session to target specific muscle groups and increase your chances of developing the ripped body that you have been looking to gain.

## Bikram Yoga

Nowadays a hugely popular trend, Bikram Yoga has suddenly gain prominence due to the heavy promotion it has received by renowned celebrities. It has been cited as the reason why Tom Cruise and George Clooney look like they have had elixir from the fountain of youth.

Superman does it and so does Batman. By that I mean, Henry Cavill and Ben Affleck respectively. And so does James Bond, Daniel Craig.

For men that's a bonus attraction. Since it goes to show how this aspect of yoga carries male friendly, masculine features.

Bikram Yoga is named after Yogi Bikram Choudhary who founded it. It is said to be a hard workout instead of meditation and breathing exercises. It focuses on the physical aspect of yoga.

It is done in a room that is heated for stretching safely as the heat loosens up the muscles, and for detoxification through sweat. The yoga poses are the same everywhere. Classes consist of the same twenty-six poses and stretches.

The temperature is kept up to a hundred or hundred and five degrees with approximately forty percent humidity levels. Expect to sweat buckets. It sounds hot, but combined with body heat and when you actually are immersed in the routine, it doesn't actually feel that hot.

Each training session goes on for ninety minutes or so.

Bikram yoga incorporates the working of every muscles, ligament, joint, and bone and is extremely helpful with avoiding injuries. It works on glands, such as thyroid, and hence aims to speed up metabolism, and balance blood sugar levels. Also there's major weight loss.

Other than that it is great with building mental strength, it gives clarity and energy. It is helpful with jetlag and maintaining healthy sleeping habits. It increases productivity, reduces stress and is good with anger management since there are a lot of breathing and balancing exercises involved.

Bikram Yoga classes are not that expensive. They do not require specific outfits or equipment. It is recommended that one does not eat at least an hour or two before a class and drink lots of water.

Yoga is a great way to tackle belly fat and crank up the body function. It increases co-ordination, balance and blood oxygen, while speeding up metabolism and thinning fat.

The most important thing it does is to strengthen muscle and access to muscle fibers. It helps with hormone control, nervous system and stress reduction. It manages your heart rate and brings about a significant decrease in risks of cardiovascular diseases.

It is not surprising that it has become so popular with celebrities and athletes.

*Andrew Creager*

# Chapter 28
# Effective Yoga Poses

Yoga poses have a lot to do with breathing and control. Inhaling, exhaling, and retaining balance are all part of a yoga routine. It is beneficial for both men and women. Men usually dismiss it as being feminine but it is actually very helpful with strengthening core muscles and building body shape.

Here are some of the most effective yoga poses:

### -Mountain (Tadasana)

Simple and effective, it increases the blood flow to the lower body and helps build a solid foundation. It improves flexibility and works with the inner thigh and core area.

How to do it: Stand with the big toes touching and heels slightly apart. Balance the weight evenly on your feet and lift up, like an arched movement. Adjust the thigh muscles slightly to lift up the kneecaps, but avoid locking your knees.

## -Tree (Vrksasana)

It strengthens the abdomen muscles and strengthens the calves and thighs.

How to do it: Shift your weight towards the right foot, pressing it firmly on to the floor. Bend the left leg at the knee and place the sole of the left foot on your inner right thigh, in a triangular angle. Point the toes toward the floor.

Place your palms together in front of your chest and keep your weight centered over the left foot. Press the right knee back while keeping your hips parallel to the front of the room. Release the foot and repeat on the other side.

## -Standing forward bend (Uttasana)

It helps with breathing, steadiness, and maintaining balance.

How to do it: It's almost like simple bending. Start as you would for a mountain pose. Bend forward at the hips. Relax your head and neck.

Ease up the shoulders and let your arms hang loosely. Place your palms or fingertips on the floor beside or slightly in front of your feet.

## -Warrior (Virabhadarasana 1)

This pose also helps stretch the calves, thighs, and chest muscles. It strengthens the lungs and shoulders as well.

How to do it: Step your right foot forward and lift your arms overhead. Turn the left foot to an angle of forty to sixty degrees to the left. Bend your right knee until it is over the ankle. Bring the hips parallel to the front of the room.

Arch your upper back in a slow movement and lift your chest up towards the ceiling. Press your palms together. If unable to do that, just keep your hands apart at a shoulder width with your palms facing each other.

Look forward or up at your thumbs. When done, step the right foot back. Repeat on the other side.

## -Downward Facing Dog (Adho Mukha Svanasana)

Much like the others, this pose also focuses on

strengthening lower body resistance and controlling breathing.

How to do it: Start on your hands and knees. Press your hands firmly on to the floor, with index fingers pointing to the front. Then as you exhale, lift your knees off the floor, keeping them slightly bent. Press your heels down toward the floor and your thighs back to straighten your legs.

Keep pressing the base of your index fingers into the floor and lift. The arms should move along with the shoulders. When done, drop your knees to the floor.

## -High Lunge (Crescent Pose)

This helps with the arms and stretching while also making your legs work harder to retain balance.

How to do it: As you exhale, step your left foot forward between your hands, keep the left knee over the ankle and your feet hip width apart.

Now when you inhale, lift your torso upright and bring your arms out to the side and overhead.

Press back through your right heel and lift up through the

torso. Repeat on the other side.

## -Boat (Navasana)

This pose is good for abs building and making shoulder muscles stronger.

How to do it: Start by being seated with your legs extended in front of you. Press your hands into the floor just behind the hips, pointing your fingers forward. Lean back slightly and lift up through your chest to prevent the back from bucking or rounding.

As you exhale, bend your knees and lift your feet off the floor until your thighs are at a forty-five degree angle from the floor. Straighten your legs slowly. When you feel stable, lift your arms off the floor and bring them out in front of you, parallel to the floor with the palms facing each other.

## -Locust (Salabhasana)

It is a challenging pose and it aims to work the upper body and lower body muscles. While stretching the thighs and leg muscles, it also works upon the chest, arms, and neck.

How to do it: Lie on your belly with your forehead touching

the floor and your hands by your hips, palms facing up. Point your big toes toward each other and slightly roll the thighs inward. Exhale and lift your head, chest, arms, and legs off the floor.

Rest your weight on your belly, lower ribs, and pelvis. As you inhale, lengthen your spine by stretching your head forward and your legs backward. Stretch back through the fingertips while keeping your arms parallel to the floor. Look down or move slightly forward to avoid crunching your neck backwards. Ease up as you exhale again.

## -Bridge (Setu Bandha Sarvangansana)

It stretches the front body along with spine and rib cage.

How to do it: Lie on your back with the arms at your sides. Bend your knees and bring your heels close to your buttocks, with the feet about hip width apart. As you exhale, push your feet and arms into the floor and lift your hips toward the ceiling. Keep your thighs parallel as your lift. Lace your fingers with each other beneath the pelvis and stretch your arms toward the feet.

## -Reclining Big Toe Pose (Supta Padangusthasana)

It is amazing for the hamstrings and hips and calves. If done the right way, it will even help make the knees stronger.

How to do it: Lie on your back. When exhaling, bend the left knee and pull it toward your chest. Keep the other leg pressed firmly onto the floor while pushing the right heel away. Hold a strap or a rope in both hands and loop it around the middle of your left foot. As you inhale, straighten your left leg slowly toward the ceiling.

Move your hands up the holder until your arms are straight, while pressing your shoulders into the floor. Once your left leg is straight, adjust the left thigh slightly and pull the foot towards the head to increase the stretch. Stay there for one to three minutes.

Then lower the left leg slowly towards the ground, keeping the right thigh pressed into the floor.

Carry on until the left leg is a few inches off the floor. Work the foot forward until it is in line with your shoulders. Inhale with your leg back to vertical. Lower the leg and repeat on the other side.

## -Sun Salutation o('Surya Namaskar')

It might be difficult to believe but a simple 'Namaste' while sitting cross legged or standing up can be a full body workout. It spurs weight reduction, stretches the spine, and increases the oxygen flow to the body.

It not only stimulates mental strength but also works towards the detoxification of the body.

These yoga poses are extremely beneficial for the body. But each of them comes with their precautions. Don't lean at awkward angles, follow the exercise properly, and keep sharp or harmful objects away from your position.

It is imperative that you know your body's condition before you attempt any of these. High blood pressure patients or people with any shoulder, knee, or neck injuries and sprains should stay away or only attempt under the supervision of a trained therapist.

For a better understanding, watch videos and consult Yoga specialists on how to best apply your body to the exercise.

# Conclusion

This book is meant to be a comprehensive guide to developing a ripped body. Unlike most books that are aimed at people who are already fitness nuts, this book is aimed at the average couch potato who wants to change their life and become a healthier, happier, well defined body.

I want everyone to enjoy the world of fitness, but I want them to do it in a safe, effective way that includes the proper preparation, the proper form, the proper nutrition, and the proper hydration. In order to develop the perfect body, you must be well prepared mentally and have a thorough understanding of what your body expects from you in order to become successful at your chosen exercise program.

The more you understand your body, and the experience of

exercise, the better you can plan your exercise routine, your diet, and your lifestyle.

Working out is not some mystical or strange experience that is difficult to get into the habit of. All it takes is a little dedication on your part and some excitement to really start shaping the way your body looks. While I have listed out many different muscle groups for you to work out and some exercises to go along with them, I want to encourage you to pair them up. Keep your leg day separate, but go ahead and make some combinations. Back and triceps go well together as do shoulders and biceps. Whatever you do, just make sure that you're hitting all of your muscle groups in a five to six day routine.

But after you've hit your days consecutively, make sure you take a rest day. One of the crucial aspects about training is letting your body heal from all the damage you've done to it and let it recharge and rebuild. If you're giving yourself ample time to rebuild and to reestablish the muscle that you have broken down, you're going to recognize better results and better gains all along the way.

However, before I mentioned all of this wonderful

information about muscle groups and how to target them effectively, I spoke to you about some important reminders before getting started. I would like to revisit those, as they're super crucial for your success. One of the things I want to remind you of is form or the general condition of your body. Your form is going to save your body from serious injuries and extensive muscle damage. You want to build up habits that you can have for years to come and the right form is going to foster that growth and that potential inside of you. Without it, you're looking at hurting yourself within the year. Play safe and make sure that your decisions are going to build you up and not tear you down.

Next, let's have a chat about nutrition and supplements. There are a lot of supplements out there on the market, but ones that I will only truly endorse are Creatine and a multivitamin. It's tried and true and it's going to help you burn fat and sculpt muscle, which is what you're looking for in this book. Apart from that, all you really need is a healthy diet. With a healthy diet, your workouts are going to give you the most gains that you're looking for. A lot of people try to completely overhaul their lives or try some weird diet, but I'm here to tell you to make subtle, but continual changes to your diet. Find what's healthy that you love and work from there. Build up your palette and grow with the experiences. If you can build a lifestyle that really fosters to your needs and interests that isn't bringing you down, you can go a long way.

Finally, be dedicated to what it is you're doing. You're making a life altering decision right now and whether you go to the gym and have an amazing workout or just an okay one, the only thing that matters is that you go! Getting there is crucial, so make your schedule and stick with it. Now, let's turn that life of yours around and get to work! Best of luck.

www.ingramcontent.com/pod-product-compliance
Lightning Source LLC
Chambersburg PA
CBHW071349280526
45787CB00001B/263